ADVANCE PRAISE FOR

The Myth of the Perfect Girl

"An essential book . . . *The Myth of the Perfect Girl* challenges both girls and the adults who care about them to deeply reflect on the most important issues girls will face as they reach their full potential."

—Rosalind Wiseman, author of *Queen Bees and Wannabes*

"As our society grapples with who we want and need females and males to grow up to be, it is no surprise that our girls and boys are confused about what is expected of them. *The Myth of the Perfect Girl* dives deep into how this is unnerving our girls. A must-read for all parents, educators, psychologists, and girls themselves."

—Dr. Louann Brizendine, founder/director of UCSF Women's Mood and Hormone Clinic and author of *The Female Brain* and *The Male Brain*

"A smart, funny, and engaging study on how to give girls the tools to figure out what they really want—and how to get it. A must-read for girls, mothers, educators, and anybody who wants to understand half the population."

—Susan Shapiro, author of *Unhooked: How to Quit Anything* and *Only as Good as Your Word*

"Many seemingly disconnected forces in society are placing unfair burdens on girls growing up today, as well as on their parents. Gratefully, Ana Homayoun poignantly spells out what's going on, how it's affecting our girls, and how grownups can help them negotiate the minefields. Everyone who cares about the well-being of girls should read *The Myth of the Perfect Girl*."

—Diane E. Levin, PhD, professor of education at Wheelock College and coauthor of *So Sexy So Soon*

continued . . .

"Whether you're the parent of an adolescent girl or a savvy young woman yourself, the insights in this book could just change your outlook—and make the turbulent teen years a little less of a pressure cooker. Ana Homayoun is the counselor, expert, and friend every parent—and girl—needs."

—Michele Borba, EdD, author of *The Big Book of Parenting Solutions*

"Offering fresh insights and vivid examples, Ana Homayoun makes sense of the enormous pressures facing girls today. More important, she shows what parents and educators can do to help girls navigate these turbulent years with confidence and purpose. A great addition to the field."

—Michael Gurian, author of *The Wonder of Girls*

PRAISE FOR

That Crumpled Paper Was Due Last Week

"Ana Homayoun gets it! Combining an extraordinary feel for what boys face in schools these days with an enormously shrewd, practical sets of tips on how to get organized and excel, this book hits a homerun. All parents and teachers as well as students (yes, I think girls could find it useful, too!) will find that this book makes school less of a struggle and more of a pleasure. Brief, to the point, and clear, this book is an invaluable, unique tool."

—Edward Hallowell, MD, author of
Super Parenting for ADD and *Driven to Distraction*

"Filled with practical advice for the parents of disorganized boys (and that's an awful lot of young boys), Ana Homayoun's *That Crumpled Paper Was Due Last Week* teaches us how to help our sons navigate through a school environment that is less than kind to distracted and disorganized young men."

—Madeline Levine, PhD, author of *The Price of Privilege*

THE MYTH OF THE
Perfect Girl

Helping Our Daughters Find
Authentic Success and Happiness
in School and Life

Ana Homayoun

A PERIGEE BOOK

A PERIGEE BOOK
Published by the Penguin Group
Penguin Group (USA) Inc.
375 Hudson Street, New York, New York 10014, USA
Penguin Group (Canada), 90 Eglinton Avenue East, Suite 700, Toronto, Ontario M4P 2Y3, Canada
(a division of Pearson Penguin Canada Inc.) • Penguin Books Ltd., 80 Strand, London WC2R 0RL,
England • Penguin Ireland, 25 St. Stephen's Green, Dublin 2, Ireland (a division of Penguin
Books Ltd.) • Penguin Group (Australia), 707 Collins Street, Melbourne, Victoria 3008, Australia
(a division of Pearson Australia Group Pty Ltd.) • Penguin Books India Pvt. Ltd., 11 Community
Centre, Panchsheel Park, New Delhi—110 017, India • Penguin Group (NZ), 67 Apollo Drive,
Rosedale, Auckland 0632, New Zealand (a division of Pearson New Zealand Ltd.) • Penguin Books,
Rosebank Office Park, 181 Jan Smuts Avenue, Parktown North 2193, South Africa • Penguin China,
B7 Jaiming Center, 27 East Third Ring Road North, Chaoyang District, Beijing 100020, China

Penguin Books Ltd., Registered Offices: 80 Strand, London WC2R 0RL, England

While the author has made every effort to provide accurate telephone numbers, Internet addresses,
and other contact information at the time of publication, neither the publisher nor the author assumes any
responsibility for errors, or for changes that occur after publication. Further, the publisher does not have any
control over and does not assume any responsibility for author or third-party websites or their content.

First edition: January 2013

Library of Congress Cataloging-in-Publication Data

Homayoun, Ana.
The myth of the perfect girl : helping our daughters find authentic success and happiness in school and life /
Ana Homayoun.
pages   cm
Includes bibliographical references and index.
ISBN: 978-0-399-53771-4
1. Daughters.   2. Girls.   3. Parenting.   4. Parenting—Religious aspects.   I. Title.
HQ777.H6646   2013
306.874—dc23   2012036341

PRINTED IN THE UNITED STATES OF AMERICA

10   9   8   7   6   5   4   3   2   1

This book describes the real experiences of real people. The author has disguised the identities of
some, and in some instances created composite characters, but none of these changes has affected
the truthfulness and accuracy of her story. Penguin is committed to publishing works of
quality and integrity. In that spirit, we are proud to offer this book to our readers;
however, the story, the experiences, and the words are the author's alone.

Most Perigee books are available at special quantity discounts for bulk purchases for
sales promotions, premiums, fund-raising, or educational use. Special books, or book
excerpts, can also be created to fit specific needs. For details, write: Special Markets,
Penguin Group (USA) Inc., 375 Hudson Street, New York, New York 10014.

ALWAYS LEARNING   PEARSON

To M. Miller,
with gratitude for your grace, wisdom,
and humor as both a mentor and a friend.

To all the girls who see themselves within the pages of this book,
I wish you a lifetime filled with personal happiness,
authenticity, and contentment.

||||||||||||||||||||||||

CONTENTS

|||||||||||||||||||||||||||

Contents

Contents

11. Conclusion: Implementing the Strategies 264

Remember the Importance of Attitude
It's Okay to Outsource
Any Day Is a Good Day to Start
Sample Six-Step Strategy

This book is about my work with preteen and teenage girls as an educational consultant and coach in schools and in private practice. Throughout these pages, I do my best to tell the personal stories about girls and their families. I have changed their names and the identifying details of their lives to protect their privacy. In some cases, I created composites based on experiences and stories of students and families with whom I worked. I hope that every preteen and teenage girl can find themselves within the pages of this book, and that every parent can find a story or experience that they themselves can relate to. Any resemblance to a particular preteen or teenage girl, however, is merely coincidental.

The Paradox of Girls' Success

Why Girls, Why Now

When Natalie and I first met, she talked a mile a minute. An over-achiever in every sense of the word, she told me how she juggled water polo with student government and volunteering at the local hospital, and that her weekends were often busier than her school weeks. In the summer, she got up at six a.m. for water polo practice, often going nonstop until ten or later at night. She kept her daily schedule on her computer, neatly color coordinated and organized, with more than a few time slots that were double- or triple-booked. I am a fairly energetic person, but listening to her was starting to wear me out.

As I noticed her winding down, I asked a simple question: "What do you like to do for fun?"

After ten minutes of bubbly effusiveness, I was met with stone-cold silence. She furrowed her brow and looked at me quizzically. "What do you mean, for fun?"

"If you had a day to yourself to do whatever you wanted, what would you do?"

I had rendered her speechless, at least for the moment. "I don't have a lot of free time," she started slowly, trying to make a statement but unable to be definitive.

I pressed on, asking what she would do for fun if she had a few free moments or days—not for a résumé or obligation, but just for pleasure. Quietly, she recoiled—she was a senior in high school, with good grades in fairly challenging classes, an extracurricular activities résumé more than a mile long, but she had no idea what she liked to do for fun. She had no hobbies, and everything she was involved with had an agenda behind it; it was all about receiving another accolade or getting to some next level of achievement.

I wish I could tell you that Natalie was an anomaly, but in fact her story has become alarmingly common among the girls I listen to on a daily basis in my office.

The Big Picture

When I started working with junior high and high school students on organization, time management, and goal setting, it initially seemed that working with boys was more challenging. Trying to get a young boy to remember to write down his assignments, complete them, and turn them in on time sometimes felt like a constant struggle. At the same time, most (though not all) of the girls seemed much more compliant and eager to please—as if they had an internal motivator to please and perfect that couldn't be turned off. They would perform and perform and perform, rarely needing to be coached back into line with school expectations. Sometimes I even wondered what my role should be with girls who were so proficient at regulating themselves.

Over the past decade, I have consulted with students, parents, faculty, and administrators throughout the United States and abroad. Through my work, it has become painfully obvious that girls are facing a different set of problems—problems that are, if anything, more challenging than the kinds of issues boys face. The girls I see are exceptionally tough on themselves for even the slightest deviation from what they deem to be the social or academic norm; many take life so seriously that it is impossible for them to feel a sense of satisfaction or fulfillment. They so fearfully dread academic humiliation that they resign themselves to taking few risks in the learning process. They learn how to "work the system," as one young woman readily explained, and in doing so fail to focus on discovering their own sense of self. For most girls, it now seems to me, the real challenge is encouraging and teaching them how to identify, disengage from, and take decisive ownership of the *external* expectations they are all too often blindly obeying. In other words, girls often need to be encouraged to find their own voice, make their own decisions, and be more skeptical of all the external expectations consciously and subconsciously placed upon them.

I think it may be helpful to step back for a moment and analyze the situation broadly. It is not at all obvious why girls should be struggling as they are. In fact, by many measurable standards of achievement, girls are doing amazingly well today. In our office, we work with many girls who are driven, motivated, and inspired to go above and beyond. Many junior high and high school principals flatly acknowledge that the majority of the top students in their classes are female. Compared to their male counterparts, young women perform better on standardized tests, outnumber men in colleges and have better college graduation rates, and now frequently outearn young men in the marketplace.[1] As Jennifer Delahunty Britz, the former director of admissions and financial aid at Kenyon College, notes in her *New York Times* op-ed piece "To All the Girls I've Rejected," the demographic reality is that many colleges now find that the stats of their female applicant pool outranks their male pool and that subsequently "the standards for admission to today's most selective colleges are stiffer for women than men."[2] In the workforce, women in their mid-twenties are, on average, making more money than their male counterparts—something that would have been unheard of thirty or forty years ago.[3] (It should still be noted that recent research shows women still make about seventy-seven cents for each dollar made by men, though those statistics are frequently challenged.[4]) All of these indicators suggest a radical shift in the kinds of large-scale cultural freedoms girls and young women can now claim and exploit in both the classroom and the workplace. And yet, it is disappointing that there is still somewhat of a glass ceiling in place, as though the ultimate paradox exists: achieve, achieve, achieve, but you can probably go only so far.

There is another, less-visible level to this story. Despite these widespread advances, both girls in school and women in the world are confronted by a paradoxical consequence of these statistics of success. Even though they are moving forward in all sorts of measurable ways, they often feel, when they stop to consider their accomplishments, that their outward successes are not matched by a sense of inner fulfillment. What sometimes emerges from these moments of self-examination is a more complicated and troubling relationship: *Girls and young women feel that they are succeeding in school and that they are failing in life for the same underlying reason*—namely, they are all too good at becoming who they think others want and need them to be. Many have yet to develop their own central core and authentic sense of spirit and are consequently apt to be toppled by whatever wind passes by. No matter what they accomplish or achieve, some girls and young women feel stuck on a treadmill of never feeling good enough and feeling convinced that happiness and fulfillment will come with the next set of accomplishments or achievements or after they have gained a certain level of social attention or perceived popularity. But, as the stakes continue to rise and the achievements mount, these girls and young women become worn down and burned out, which contributes to a host of other social and emotional challenges.

How Success and Failure Are Sometimes the Same Thing

Even as girls are succeeding in remarkable ways, we (and by *we* I mean parents, educators, psychologists, peers, and even the girls themselves) are finding that more and more of them are struggling. Compared to boys, girls have higher rates of mental illnesses like depression and anxiety.[5] Research shows that girls between the ages of fifteen and twenty have more than *double* the rates of depression than that of their male counterparts.[6] Those who fulfill the criteria for a diagnosis of major depression are much more likely to also struggle with anxiety, conduct disorders, and/or addictive disorders.[7] They often grapple with eating disorders and negative body self-image. There is, as I will be mentioning throughout the book, virtually an epidemic of meanness from girls directed at girls. More than one in five girls in high school admit to have seriously considered committing suicide.[8] In general, teenage girls seem to be experiencing success and certain kinds of acute unhappiness at the same, accelerating rates. As Rachel Simmons notes in her book *The Curse of the Good Girl*, "Many of the most accomplished girls are disconnecting from the truest parts of themselves, sacrificing essential self-knowledge to the pressure of who they think they ought to be."[9]

In our achievement-oriented educational system and culture, these girls are often one step away from burnout—physically, emotionally, and socially exhausted from running after externally rewarding accomplishments, yet hungry for more substantial internal filling. In their quest to achieve external standards of perfection, they struggle to figure out what brings them personal purpose, joy, or fulfillment. Like Natalie, they have a long list of extraordinary accomplishments but little to say about what really pleases them. And like Natalie, many of them never truly feel good enough.

I think many of us understand, intuitively, that the frenzied accumulation of winnings is not going to lead to lasting satisfaction. My goal here is to articulate the heart of girls' struggles, which is something I call *filling the box*.

Filling the Box

We often hear the phrase *think outside the box* used to describe the notion of thinking beyond the rote and normal of everyday expectations. That is, *thinking outside the box* denotes the importance of thinking differently, consciously, individually, and proactively. *Filling the box* is the metaphor I use to describe the *opposite* movement: girls' tendency to be compliant to others' expectations rather than creating and pursuing their own version of personal success and fulfillment. The idea of filling the box came to me when I was speaking to a young woman who was just about to graduate from a prestigious business school and felt utterly lost. Even though she had a job lined up, she was terrified. "As long as I have a regimented box to fill," she explained, motioning with her hands, "I am fine. But the minute I have to come up with something on my own . . ." Her voice trailed off, and she seemed utterly overwhelmed.

The image of filling someone else's box, rather than building and creating one's own, is a way of capturing how many girls and young women accept the structures of achievement and definitions of success from outside themselves. Girls are more apt to find and measure their self-worth through external validation than through internal reflection. Some of that is developmental—a young girl may look to her parents and adults for guidance, whereas an adolescent girl will naturally try to break free from parental involvement and look to her peers for approval. However, when girls and young women fail to develop their own authentic voice, spirit, and sense of personal purpose, they run the risk, by default, of simply following the lead of others. In time, these girls and young women become overly dependent on others to design, motivate, and evaluate the goals they set out to achieve.

Our school structure today, with its emphasis on exams, standardized tests, and other measurable indicators of achievement, has become a breeding ground for mirroring and box filling. Girls are able (and indeed endlessly encouraged) to study for exams, properly align their papers, and rework and revise to their heart's content. They are frequently reminded about college applications and admission standards, beginning at younger and younger ages. I cannot tell you the number of times in recent years I have had staring contests with students who show up at the office and want to know *exactly what they need to say* on the essay they're writing in order to do well. They have gotten so used to being told how to think, answer, or analyze, that being asked to come up with original ideas seems to frighten them. The too-stringent focus on results eliminates the possibility of learning from mistakes. More and more, students become passive toward the educational process because they learn that getting the right answer, rather than knowing how to think through a problem, is rewarded. I am always a little dismayed when I ask a student about how she is doing, which I mean as a general question to her overall well-being, and I receive a response that is something along the lines of, "Well, I am worried I won't get an A in math." How they feel becomes inextricably linked to how they are doing in school, and it is difficult for them to delineate otherwise.

And it's not just inside the classroom. Magazines preach ways to achieve the perfect hair, skin, and body; celebrities promote effortless perfection as a viable indicator of success. Both school and our culture at large offer countless ways for girls to follow externally set standards—how to get good grades; how to be involved extracurricularly, socially, and athletically; how to look, dress, and feel—and many girls have become so busy trying to squeeze themselves into fitting such standards they have lost touch with their own power to shape themselves and their lives.

Why Is Filling the Box a Girl Phenomenon?

Some may wonder if and how this notion of filling the box is specific to girls. It certainly feels like we live in a generally achievement-oriented culture, and that both girls and boys are struggling to keep up with rampant expectations. So why focus on girls? It's a good question, and of course it's true that most kids today are overpressured to achieve, whether in sports, academics, socially, or myriad other ways. But I do think, based on over a decade of working with school-age students and young adults, as well as the research from many other child development experts, that the pressure to perform hits girls in particularly damaging ways and does so for three main reasons. First is the crucial fact that girls tend to be natural pleasers and want to do things the way they think they are supposed to. Despite their historically increasing independence, girls are still, to an extent that boys typically are not, eager to please their teachers, friends, parents, and cultural heroes by unquestioningly following directions. I once calmly and quietly told a young girl in my office that she did not have to apologize so frequently—she would say "sorry" if she got a math problem wrong or if she made a careless error in grammar on a paper. Over the course of an hour, I must have heard "sorry!" almost a hundred times. When I encouraged her to stop apologizing for not understanding material she was in the process of learning, she looked a bit terrified at what she must have interpreted as shocking criticism and then apologized for apologizing too much.

As a result, given an extraordinarily surface- and bottom-line driven environment like modern American society, girls are almost psychosocially predisposed to fail to develop their intrinsic motivations and personal interests. The flip side to their greater natural responsibility is their weaker tendency to go against the grain. This is why the filling-the-box problem extends beyond merely academic concerns. Modern society is ever more eager to judge people by their conformity to templates across a whole range of behaviors: schools test more, advertisers airbrush more blatantly, TV blares more loudly to a lower common denominator, and, most recent, social media networks can often perform a kind of hyperpervasive, instant social norming. Girls are typically ahead of their male peers in mastering some of these diverse media but are also more likely to be influenced by them in forming their expectations for themselves. Many of these girls give off the perception that everything is perfect on the outside, when, in reality, they are waging a personal nightmare on the inside.

The second reason for their greater vulnerability to box filling is that adolescent girls and young women (as well as many older women) tend to be much more relationship oriented than their male peers. This is related to but importantly different from the first point. Girls want to please the authorities around them and do what the authorities think they should do, but girls also derive an enormous amount of their self-worth from their relationships, and therefore put a lot of energy not only into meeting expectations but also into constructing friendships and monitoring their positions in them. Put more simply, girls care deeply about their relationships and what other people think of them. So not only do they struggle to develop an authentic sense of what they enjoy but they are also overly dependent on approval from peers and do not easily understand who they are socially. Indeed, research reveals that girls who have negative perceptions of their own peer interpersonal relationships and school experiences (that is, girls who don't have good relationships with their peers and who don't like school) are more likely to experience negative mental health effects.[10] Indeed, a middle school girl's entire day can be ruined because a so-called friend looked at her oddly or she didn't receive an invitation to the right party. I have seen girls who are doing well in school and are leaders within their community sit in my office nearly paralyzed by the fear that they won't get a date for the prom or become worked up by drama about who will be in a certain party bus or limo for a certain dance. They want to be liked and to have friends—it's natural and there's nothing wrong with it. But it means that in a hypersocialized, achievement-obsessed world (as I discuss in more detail in Chapter 1), these girls are more likely to constrain themselves to others' cues to conform.

And finally, girls begin puberty earlier and often mature faster than do boys, and their earlier physical and emotional maturity frequently leaves them trying to figure out their place in the world without the guidance and encouragement needed to develop their own sense of personal purpose. Our schools and social systems today tend to overlook emphasizing individualized development in favor of overarching achievement and self-promotion, and girls can struggle to develop their own values and individualized belief systems. Encouraging critical thinking and character development has become virtually nonexistent in schools where priority is put on numbers-based performance. Consequently, girls begin to follow the preset external standards of excellence readily touted in schools, magazines, media, and elsewhere in hopes that they will gain the inner fulfillment and satisfaction they so desperately desire.

Pleasing Everyone but Themselves

For years, I helped students organize their college application process. My philosophy had always been to help them figure out who they are and what they enjoyed and then to help them manage their own process, including teaching them how to schedule their time so the whole procedure was less overwhelming. My hope was that they are able to begin developing their own voice and sense of themselves before going off on their own for the first time in their lives. That was the hope, but increasingly I find myself working with girls who had a lot of work to do *undoing* the very patterns of thought they'd strenuously built up over years of living up to external standards of social and academic success.

One recent spring day, in my usual practice of having an introductory meeting with high school juniors, I had the alarming experience of back-to-back meetings with four different girls who seemed identical. They had strong grades, took rigorous classes, achieved top SAT scores, and were active in their schools and local communities. Their extracurricular activities were interchangeable: Two played club volleyball, another was on a traveling soccer team that practiced twenty hours a week, and the last one was being recruited to play field hockey at the collegiate level. But what struck me most was that no matter what they were doing and how much they were doing, they were always worried that they weren't doing enough. Not only that, they each looked like they could have used an extra thirty or so hours of sleep. Two of them spoke with the slowness that only exhaustion brings, and the other two came in with extra-large caffeinated drinks.

As each meeting progressed, I could sense these girls' anxiety bubbling up. They had spent countless hours talking with friends, parents, and other well-meaning adults about getting into a really good school. In school and in life, they had taken few, if any real risks—and the risks they did take were calculated and ends-oriented. Not one of them could think of the last time she had an afternoon to do something frivolous and fun. They'd overanalyzed and overthought, and they had spent their high school years compulsively filling the box, hoping they were doing everything right to get to the next level of achievement, where, it was all too obvious, the endless chase would begin once more. I have learned to be far more worried about these overprogrammed students than for most of the kids who come into my office struggling with disorganization.

The consequences here are extremely broad and very deep. One of the lessons of modern life is that we have to make our own way—there are no automatic authorities to tell us what is right. We don't just follow the paths laid out for us by our class or gender or by what our parents did. And this requires self-reflection about what matters to us, if we're going to align our actions with our purposes. Without reflection, we're vulnerable to the agenda-setting whims of the many minor authorities that are propped up in our culture—from celebrities to diet-book gurus to abstract notions like "prestige" and "perfection." The problem is that girls are not often taught how to identify their deepest desires, and when they are taught, it's not early enough. Combined with their tendency to be pleasers, this puts them at risk, over years and years, of serving interests outside themselves.

The Empty Box

What results is a feeling of internal emptiness (an *empty box*) that leaves girls simply running on a treadmill of increased box filling. For many girls, the ideal of having to be perfect is an unobtainable vision that leaves them constantly thirsting for more and constantly feeling as though they are never good enough. The pursuit of real but insufficiently nourishing achievement becomes a self-perpetuating cycle: pleasing, achieving, getting, and then seeking more ways to receive external validation. Trying to assuage that emptiness, some girls become snarky and mean; they strive for performances of improbable and effortless perfection. Others resort to compensatory behaviors like food and exercise obsessions, social media addiction, drug and alcohol abuse, and emotionally unfulfilling sexual relationships to fill the emptiness. The troubling effects of this vicious circle are evident in playgrounds, classrooms, and offices all across society.

Not long ago, I was meeting with a junior high school principal and school psychologist to discuss the challenges in their seventh- and eighth-grade classes. The school psychologist brought up the problems among a group of seventh-grade girls who practiced a deep-seated meanness and snarkiness that left virtually no one unscathed. I found myself quoting a phrase I often use with students who have faced the wrath of another person's meanness: "People who are mean generally don't like themselves." It's a simple premise, really, but it gets to the heart of a lot of mean behavior, and thinking it through can change a student's perspective surprisingly quickly. I remember the first time I proposed it to a girl who had come into the office upset, supposedly over a math test, but really, as it turned out, about an acquaintance's snide remark. The girl suddenly softened when she realized that the other girl's behavior had more to do with *her* internal emptiness than anything else.

Similarly on this occasion, my observation caused both the principal and the psychologist to stop and reflect. "You're right," the principal said slowly, "I really don't think these girls like themselves at all. When you talk with them, they seem to be empty inside." The school psychologist chimed in, "Well, when you think about it, it's *easy* to see that they don't like themselves."

I agree. It wasn't surprising, and it *is* easy to see when you look for it—after all, very few self-accepting, well-adjusted individuals actively want to cause another person's misery. But I think we need to pay closer attention to what incidents like these are telling us. We need to see the epidemic of meanness, for example, for the sign it is: *whole ranges and cohorts of girls who are struggling to adjust to their own lives and developments in the face of academic and social pressures,* with no internal compass or sense of who they are. This, in the broadest sense, is the condition that I want to bring into view—girls who try to fill the emptiness by pushing ever further outside themselves: by pursuing unobtainable perfection academically or physically, by either starving or stuffing themselves, by living off the cheap thrills from putting others down, or sometimes by resigning themselves to a lack of fulfillment, becoming depressed, and withdrawing from their lives.

As I will discuss in the following chapters, these are all versions of filling the box. As these examples already suggest, my concern is that it's the darker flip side to the whole culture of achievement. Girls are encouraged to meet an array of external standards; they are in some ways predisposed to find their satisfactions in the ways they fit these kinds of measurements. Because when girls are not always readily encouraged to identify their personal interests and sense of purpose, let alone to value them, they fail to develop the spiritual or philosophical self-recognition that could anchor them when they fail, inevitably, to find themselves in yet one more outside accolade or achievement.

A few years ago, I was amazed at the number of times I had to convince girls coming into my office to calm down, relax, and try simply to find more joy. These girls made me nervous, in part because they reminded me uncomfortably of a much more hard-charging version of myself when I was their age. Today, I am less amazed than inured to the new reality. Now, I look around and see so many young women in their twenties and thirties still trying mechanically to fill their boxes— almost like robots, acting and performing but feeling like they are never good enough, racing ahead to fill their hunger, never satisfied.

But there is hope. Hard as it is, the stream of conventional success can be fought against in the direction of real pleasure and purpose. I am a firm believer in dreaming big and having wonderfully imperfect, messy, enriching lives. In working with girls, my goal is fundamentally to help them gain more self-acceptance, more self-awareness, and the ability to develop and articulate their own sense of purpose. I want to help them forge the anchor that can hold them in place when everyone else is calling for them to conform. But in order to do so, you and I, as parents and educators, and the girls themselves, need to work at promoting positive change in girls' self-perceptions. We need to replace the success treadmill so that ultimately, instead of exhausting themselves trying to fill an empty box, girls are building and expanding their own world.

|||||||||||||||||||||||

CHAPTER ONE

The Perfect Girl Myth

Why It's So Prevalent and Such a Problem

A few years ago, I was meeting with a high school senior whose boyfriend had recently broken up with her. Noticeably distraught, she tried to sneak a peek at her cell phone every two minutes until I finally took the phone and put it on the top of my bookshelf for the remainder of our session. She was deeply embarrassed about how the breakup was being perceived—by her friends, by anyone who might be surfing her Facebook page and realize that she was no longer in a relationship, indeed, by all the people out there in the world who could be electronically witnessing her humiliation. The prospect of having to defend herself from the potential onslaught of unwelcome attention was overwhelming: She was crying in my office and unsuccessfully trying to focus on studying for final exams; and she was simultaneously trying to appear calm and totally unable to keep herself from scrambling around cyberspace trying to manage the crisis.

What's Different Now?

Parents often ask me, "What's different now? Haven't girls always faced problems like these? Aren't they always going through some emotional catastrophe? Indeed, isn't adolescence an emotional catastrophe in itself? Isn't going through this and growing out of it just the way girls are?"

My answer is yes, part of being a girl and growing up is learning to struggle with upheaval and disappointment and change: being painfully attentive to it, sometimes too good at analyzing it in detail, and finally learning lessons and moving on. Some of this has always led some girls to conform themselves into conventional, unfulfilling pursuits.

But our time is very different for a number of reasons, reasons that make the challenges facing girls more urgent and explosive than ever before. A series of modern and hypermodern developments that we think of as in part defining our current world are combining to bring the pressures of compliance and empty success to a new pitch of intensity. Situations and behaviors that previously might have passed innocuously by as the way things are have been magnified under the conditions of modern life. I frequently see girls becoming unglued at receiving a less than stellar grade on a paper or test or feeling as though they are never going to be successful in life after experiencing what should seem like a minor setback or rejection.

The distraught breakup anecdote opening this chapter illustrates the scope of these changes. The point of the story is not the breakup itself, but the fact that the crisis in this girl's life was terribly, even incapacitatingly, intensified by its exposure to a whole wide world of potential participants. It is almost as though there were *two* breakups: the familiar, human-scale one with tears and laments and self-analysis and then an utterly new, explosively magnified one reaching out across the Internet and an entire social universe, which subjected this one girl, at least in her mind, to the seeming censure of the world. Today, the Internet can make something that is hard enough to deal with privately ever more daunting by bringing problems to public attention. In the more public situation, a girl can find herself focusing on how others view her rather than focusing on how she is dealing with the issue at hand.

We have not properly prepared our girls to succeed authentically in such an environment. And until we get a handle on the nature of the changes involved, we will not be in a position to help girls resist and redirect the pressures and temptations to which they are increasingly falling prey.

There are five main structural reasons for the rise of the box-filling epidemic. Understanding some of this background, I hope, will put us all in a better position to appreciate the extent of and diagnose the risks of the current perils.

Reason 1: Our Changing Academic Landscape

As an experiment, I often ask parents of the girls I work with to reflect on what they did when they were young to prepare for the SAT, a test that is still one of the primary exams for college admissions. Most admit they did nothing more than get a good night's sleep, eat breakfast, and show up on time. If they were lucky, they remembered to bring a calculator and some number 2 pencils. Today, it's an entirely different world. Many girls (and boys) know not only their friends' scores but also, thanks to a thriving industry of books and articles devoted to the subject, the average scores of entrants into nearly every college in the country. Culturally, the importance of testing and its associated metrics has been exaggerated out of proportion, such that test prep is now a nearly billion-dollar industry. In many schools, standardized testing starts in the elementary grades (or earlier). And the same parents who were so nonchalant in their own cases are now spending thousands of dollars helping their kids prepare for standardized tests; students are devoting hundreds of hours to taking practice tests, learning vocabulary with flashcards, and mastering the art of guessing by elimination.

Although this kind of frenzied focus on testing is, I think, quite familiar, we don't often acknowledge how close it comes to being truly problematic. Most of us have no idea of the extremes to which this anxiety runs. In 2011, prosecutors in Long Island, New York, cracked down on a SAT cheating scandal when a young man, Samuel Eshaghoff, was paid as much as several thousand dollars to impersonate and fraudulently take the SAT test for at least fifteen students who desperately wanted to score well in their quest for college admissions. According to *New York Times* reporters Jenny Anderson and Peter Applebome, "It was common knowledge at some of the nation's most prestigious high schools that if you had the money, you could find someone with a sharper vocabulary and a surer grasp of geometry to fill in the blanks for you."[1] Not long thereafter, a senior admissions official at Claremont McKenna, a well-respected liberal arts college in southern California, resigned after confessing to routinely inflating the reported SAT scores of entering freshmen in attempts to present a more impressive picture of the college's "selectivity."[2] Clearly, even colleges are worried about SAT scores. And given the depths of the testing chaos, is it any wonder that many students consciously and subconsciously measure themselves and their self-worth by these numbers?

One girl I worked with summarized the effect of this emphasis on numerical performance: "I sometimes feel like little more than the sum of my numbers." She went on to describe her feeling that her identity was tied to her SAT scores, AP scores, GPA, and, somewhat humorously, her time running the mile in PE class.

In the past twenty or thirty years, "standards of excellence" as reflected by expectations of achievement in schools have increased exponentially. But I put that phrase in quotation marks because I am not at all sure that actual standards have changed very much or that we really know what we mean by the idea. And yet, we are all doing a lot more talking about high standards and about sticking to them and demanding that our kids meet them.

What can get lost in this concentration on high standards is the focus on the individual student's interests and needs. Teaching and excellence—and teaching excellence—like most things that matter, are always very specific. There is little evidence, for example, that doing more homework improves student understanding very much. At a certain point, it turns into busywork, or a nightly marathon whose goal is finishing rather than figuring anything out.

When and how did we get to this place, in the last few decades, where *schooling* has become, in many cases, synonymous with *testing*? Certainly various legislative actions have contributed. But, even aside from the bias of school policy, and stemming perhaps from a similar obsession with "officially authorized" learning, there is also a palpable increase in blatant achievement orientation: a nonstop competition that begins at birth among many overzealous parents. The ubiquity of advertising, the continual drive to commercialize even the most wholesome goods, and the technology-enabled ease of comparing oneself to anyone from any kind of background or accomplishment have all conspired to turn an entire generation of parents into Ivy League wannabes. And so, it's not simply high school students who are experiencing stress about the college application process; the pressure is being felt by parents who feel they will be judged by their child's school choices. This pressure is also being felt at younger and younger ages, as sixth graders sometimes confide to me their fears over whether they will get into a good college, even though their ideas of what that means are hazy at best.

At a local public school near my office, there is a math placement test given to sixth graders that determines which math class students are placed in for the seventh grade. Many parents believe that how their eleven- or twelve-year-old performs on this math placement test will strongly affect the colleges he or she can get into—imagine the *pressure*. Some parents schedule extensive private tutoring so the child can pass the test for the desired class. Depending on the child, this can help or hurt. As Berkeley psychology professor Stephen Hinshaw notes in his book *The Triple Bind*, it can be unbelievably damaging to force a child to perform developmental tasks before he or she is ready.[3] In essence, children learn best (faster, more lastingly, and with greater enthusiasm) at the rate that is developmentally appropriate for them and allows them to feel in charge of the material.

I have often seen a young girl who is doing just fine in the regular math group and feeling confident about her math skills pushed into entering the higher group. Too often, the confidence gained from mastery of the developmentally appropriate material, and that was flowing virtuously into all the rest of the student's classes, is burst when she begins to struggle in the new setting. Suddenly, I start to hear refrains of "I'm not good at math" or "I'm not a math person."

It can make for a long and excruciating story of unnecessary alienation. Ironically, the parents who wouldn't let their daughter miss a chance to excel are the very ones who set her down a path of missed opportunities for real growth. The girl who was once swimming along comfortably is now flapping around in the deep end, barely holding on for dear life. Homework becomes overwhelming, and math tests are anxiety ridden. Big holes open up in her basic grasp of concepts. Years later, in high school and beyond, math becomes even more difficult, and fluency with the ideas is harder to fake or finesse, and the constant struggle is demoralizing. The end result is that she may lose interest in math altogether, in part because she is driven to conclude that her innate ability is subpar. Had she continued at her own pace and received good, focused instruction, perhaps math would have remained a source of strength, and perhaps she would have found her way into the higher class when she was ready to tackle it. As child psychologist and school counselor Judy Rothenberg often exclaims in regard to math preparation, "I tell parents it doesn't matter when they get it. It just matters that they get it."[4]

School administrators often note the increasing number of parents of kindergartners who want to know what types of colleges the high school seniors in the district or private K–12 school are getting into. For many of them, acceptance to certain well-regarded colleges is from the very beginning the overriding measure of their kids' success.

In the past few decades, college admissions rates have become dramatically low at some of the nation's most well-known colleges, adding to the panic of many parents and students. For instance, in 2012, several colleges hit new lows in admission rates—with more than a few highly selective schools accepting less than 10 percent of applicants— meaning that nine out of every ten applicants were rejected.[5] And even though there are still hundreds of colleges and universities that accept well over 50 percent of their applicants for undergraduate admission, there has become this intense propensity to focus on coveting the elusive acceptance. At the same time, college tuition has increased at a shocking rate. In his *Wall Street Journal* article titled "College: Big Investment or Big Risk?," columnist Jack Hough notes data from the U.S. Labor Department showing that college tuition and fees have increased 184 percent over the past twenty years, adjusted for inflation, even though the rise in salaries for recent graduates has increased only 9 percent.[6] The decreased likelihood of admissions and increased cost of attendance can add to the stress of social and economic challenges, by which young students can feel more pressure to be finished products and have set career paths to justify the strain of rising college tuition. At the same time, some parents start to think that if they are going to pay that much for college, it had better be a good school.

All of these developments conspire to reverse the traditional perspective on childhood. Kids, especially high school students, are less likely to be regarded as involved in a valuable process of learning, creative exploration, and personal development that helps them become active makers of their own futures. Or if the process is valued, it's immediately subordinated to the greater value of the success it's supposed to lead to. Activities deemed to be fun and play are now denigrated as unimportant unless they support the success agenda behind them. The development of personal character and values, which requires thoughtful processing and room to learn from mistakes, has been thwarted to a role of less importance than tangible achievements. Future attainments—test scores, college admissions, and later on jobs, positions, and awards—are increasingly seen as the ultimate ends toward which the education of children is just one important means. The résumé is driving the education rather than the other way around.

It's important to emphasize how new this culture of achievement is. People have always striven for the best, of course, but the *single-minded focus* with which this end-results perspective attacks and upends the system of education and its breadth across the culture are new, and girls, who are more prone to buying into its temporary rewards, are especially at risk. This brings me back to the empty box syndrome I described in the introduction. This change comes at a cost, and one of the principal areas being made to pay is the emotional well-being of girls. It's a paradoxical fact that the kind of streamlined expectations underlying the modern embrace of standardized testing and much of modern curricular design have been both a blessing and a curse for girls. Many child-development experts argue that schools today are seemingly tailor-made for girls' style of learning, while being far from optimal for boys. My first book, *That Crumpled Paper Was Due Last Week*, focuses on how boys struggle to keep up in today's schools. Girls, by contrast, seem as though they have never been doing better, at least as far as numbers are concerned.

But this change also funnels girls directly down into all the dangers of the achievement trap. Girls tend to be better at following directions and at being responsive, caught up, and organized with their work, but they also fail to question the terms of the success to which they are implicitly agreeing. Even girls who struggle with organization and time management (as many do, especially as we expect so much more of them so much earlier) generally zero in on what they need to do to get through the class in question. In the longer run, the profile that some modern schools favor—the rule-following, stick-to-the-assignment, compliant producer of measurable results—keeps girls from succeeding in deeper, more far-ranging ways. And so, even though our schools have been productive in breaking girls free of traditional limits, we are now seeing that many girls are failing to grow into the thoughtful, self-reflective learners, thinkers, and innovators that our world wants and needs.

Reason 2: Getting Older Younger
EARLY-ONSET PUBERTY AND THE SEXUALIZATION OF GIRLS

Between the sixth and seventh grade, Rania grew three inches. Suddenly, her favorite jeans weren't just too short but also too tight in the waist and the thighs—dashing her hopes that her jeans' life span could be extended as capris. She had developed a bit of a chest, which was not enough to really warrant the use of a bra, but she definitely felt more confident with one on at all times. Which made the day that she forgot to pack a bra to wear after morning swim practice the Worst.Day.Ever. Everything seemed to spiral downward—the lack of a bra; the map test on the Middle East, during which she drew a blank and forgot three of the countries and capitals; and the lunch drama with her supposed best friend, Samantha, who had begun hanging out with a new group of girls and had let everyone at lunch know about Rania's bra-less day. Her classmates kept coming up and rubbing her back and making comments, and Rania felt as if she were crawling out of her own skin. By the end of school that day, she had half-decided that the best course of action would be to move to a new town.

Hitting puberty is a bit like going through menopause. Pubescent girls, quite like menopausal women, never know how or when their hormones are going to shift and how these changes are going to affect them. As a result, girls' behavioral patterns during puberty are wildly unpredictable. Most parents can remember their daughter having a complete and utter meltdown over something seemingly innocuous that has suddenly become overwhelming. Maybe a boy looked at her weirdly in the hallway, and it makes her think everyone hates her and leads her to believe everyone is talking about her. Almost anything can seem to set her off. But the effect of hormones shouldn't be minimized as merely "typical"; the lack of control she feels in this aspect of her life may push her to seek control elsewhere—especially in school, where she spends the majority of her waking hours. She may compensate, for example, by becoming hyperorganized and striving to be the best student she can be, by strictly defining what success means and pegging it to certain accomplishments or status in her athletic or social life, or by placing restrictions and limitations on her food choices.

What makes the process of puberty and hormones even more challenging is that girls are developmentally pretty self-focused and self-centered, so the ability to understand and empathize with the mood swings and daily drama of themselves and of others can be incredibly challenging. For girls, the here and now becomes utterly important as they attempt to regain control in their lives. Conformity and box-filling behavior may be one way of artificially reestablishing the control that seems so painfully out of reach.

Very few individuals who have gone through puberty look back at the experience with only fond memories. After all, puberty is often a time of complete upheaval, when there are so many different emotional, physical, and mental changes happening all at once. And even that one girl from homeroom who had no acne, a perfect body, and hair that was oh-so-shiny (most of us know at least one) still had to deal with the anxieties and identity crises that are part of puberty's rite of passage.

And now, the natural synchronization of this biological-cultural movement is being disrupted, or at least significantly altered. There is a rise in *precocious puberty*—that is, the start of puberty at age seven or eight years old. Girls today are, on average, entering puberty fully a year or two (and sometimes more) earlier than thirty years ago. Endocrine disruptors, which are chemicals in food and the environment that mimic female sex hormones, and rates of obesity are considered major factors in this monumental change. Precocious puberty has potentially enormous, and largely unacknowledged, consequences for the ways girls experience their own development. Although most research and analysis are still in the early stages, indications are that precocious puberty may have a negative impact on girls' long-term mental and emotional health. As Diana Zuckerman notes, "Many young girls in early elementary school are developing breasts and pubic hair at a time when they are still playing with dolls and Junior Monopoly, and are too young to understand the emotional mood swings and other symptoms of adolescence."[7]

Starting puberty early can be an incredibly disjointed experience, and although this is happening more and more, society is just starting to recognize the shift. Very few schools have proper support for these girls—for example, most elementary schools do not have feminine hygiene supplies in the school bathroom or appropriate receptacles in the stalls. For girls who are menstruating so young, this can cause further embarrassment and shame.

And it's not just the girls who begin puberty earlier who are struggling. Those who are a few steps behind, on what used to be considered a normal timetable, are also often made to feel self-conscious about their relatively later maturation. These girls may feel as though they must conform in different ways—wear more provocative clothing or show through their behavior that they are more advanced than their bodies suggest. Or they may resort to other behaviors like academic or social control or athletic or extracurricular accomplishments to compensate for feeling out of place.

In addition to the effects on girls' self-perceptions, their earlier sexual maturity makes a big difference in the way they are treated by others. Girls may or may not understand what they're feeling earlier, but it's clear that if they *look* more mature at younger ages, *other people* will happily treat them as though they were older.

What gets lost in both the biological and commercial rush to adulthood, is the safe haven of ordinary childhood. Girls who look like young women before they're ten years old results in the confusing situation of puberty overlapping with childhood. Though the research is currently limited, it's not hard to imagine that girls who look like teenagers when they are still in elementary school feel both strangely self-assured and, partly as a result, self-conscious and overwhelmed.[8] How can you feel like a grown-up if you haven't actually grown up? With bodies changing, hormones swinging, and feelings developing, these girls are prime candidates for the defensive numbness that comes from emptiness.

THE SEXUALIZATION OF GIRLS

Most parents of a preteen, tween, or teenager will acknowledge how challenging it is to find appropriate clothes for girls in this age group. At the same time that girls feel self-conscious because their minds and limbs and body parts are developing at different rates, they are pushed to wear shorter hemlines and lower necklines than ever before. Lip gloss and mascara are made in child-friendly cases, and young girls accompany their moms to the spa for manicures, pedicures, and massages—something that would have been unheard of several decades ago. We have taught a whole generation of young girls to primp, prod, wax, and flat-iron in imitation of a standard that, even for their mothers, is radically sexualized. This focus on beauty and appearance pervades our culture. It's impossible to ignore, and even those of us who may think it odd that a six-year-old has a makeup bag find ourselves tacitly accepting the new norm. In her eye-opening book *Cinderella Ate My Daughter*, Peggy Orenstein examines how makeup products and sexually revealing clothes are targeted at younger girls than ever before, with the all-too-intentional side effect that our sensibilities get warped:

> Our tolerance for hypersexualization rises without us realizing it . . .
> we get used to seeing twelve-year-olds in lip-gloss, low-slung jeans,

and crop tops that say BAD GIRL, and soon the same outfit seems
unremarkable on an eight-year-old.[9]

Candie's is a successful clothing company that targets eight- to sixteen-
year-old girls. Their clothing line and related advertisements provide a
clear window to the sexualization of girls that has become more and
more commonplace in recent years. In a typical ad, a tanned girl is
featured posing provocatively with her legs in the air, wearing short
shorts, a tank top, and wedge heels, and giving a come-hither look to
the camera. In 2012, Lea Michele, an actress whose credits include
the television show *Glee*, was named the "Candie's Girl of the Year."[10]
At twenty-five years old, she is at least a decade older than the target
audience, and her photo shoot for the ad campaign included poses that,
with only slightly less clothing, might have been mistaken for an adult
magazine photo shoot. In several pictures, she is lying on a bed of pink
satin sheets, surrounded by fur pillows, wearing short shorts or a short
skirt and platform heels. In others, she splays suggestively on a kitchen
counter or in the bathroom or in front of the closet.[11]

One particularly revealing version of this whole dynamic is the
concept of "age compression." In their book *So Sexy So Soon*, child development and media experts Diane Levin and Jean Kilbourne describe
the ways childhood has become a period of increasingly accelerated
pseudo-development. *Age compression* is the term that child-marketing
professionals use "to describe how children at ever younger ages are
doing what older children used to do."[12] Academically, we have accelerated preschools and honors-track classes that make it possible for students to take college-level coursework during their sophomore year in
high school. Socially, girls are bombarded with messages to dress and
act older to be accepted. Extracurricularly and athletically, girls face a
gnawing fear that whatever they are doing isn't enough to get that college scholarship or entrance on the Junior Olympic Development Program squad.

Girls of previous generations certainly had their own challenges, but they were, more often than not, given the opportunity to be girls. When we think of the concept of today's age compression metaphorically, as representing the general trend of change, we come closer to the heart of the matter. *Age compression* can stand for how, in this race to act and seem older earlier than ever before, the substance of self-awareness has been squeezed out. It's what is lost when actual learning and self-knowledge are replaced by usually commercialized versions of someone else's agenda.

Coupled with the increased sexualization of girls—indeed as a large part of that same objectifying message—the warped notion of beauty and health has enormously intensified the box-filling problem. When girls fix on a celebrity or media figure as a model, the chosen image has almost always been airbrushed and reshaped.[13] This produces a kind of double emptiness: Girls who already focus on outside expectations are choosing, as a guide for how to look and how to act, images that are themselves empty of substance. Even more confusing for some girls is when their mothers use extensive treatments to try to appear younger, while the girls use makeup and treatments to try to appear older. No one, it seems, can happily accept herself as she is.

> No one, it seems, can happily accept herself as she is.

Marketers are clearly focused on finding ways to sell their products, but their avid competition for consumers makes it easy for younger girls, sometimes almost accidentally, to tap into the deluge of confusing sexual imagery. Fifteen or twenty years ago, parents could much more readily filter their kids' television viewing. Now, Internet-ready phones connect adult-oriented content to whomever chooses to look and may leave girls with uncomfortable questions about how they should think and behave. Exercising the duty of parental surveillance has never been more necessary, or more difficult.

Somehow, in this modern culture, we've turned around in a circle, and girls have gotten the message that being sexy and hot is empowering. But the long-term effects of exposure to these adult, idealized images can be damaging. The American Psychological Association's Task Force on the Sexualization of Girls notes that girls who are exposed to such idealized images tend to have lower opinions of themselves and are more likely to struggle with depression and anxiety.[14] One of the most striking suggestions made by the task force is that girls' exposure to images of sexualization, in which women are depicted as sexual ornaments for others' use, may increase their *self-objectification*, by which they learn to regard themselves as objects to be used by others.

What is the cost of allowing girls to watch adult-themed movies or read sex-stuffed women's magazines or wear short shorts? It turns out that it's pretty much what you would expect: Girls who are confused about their roles, who think of themselves as primarily sexual beings, and who have been encouraged to essentially skip a childhood are trained to perceive themselves as they are perceived by others. This is box filling epitomized: *Living through yourself for others' desires and to be desired by others.*

One of the most challenging long-term implications of this sexualization of girls is the way in which boys' and girls' relationships with one another get caught up in the vicious circle. Instead of playing together in elementary school and developing collaborative friendships, young boys and girls get to know each other in an atmosphere of early sexualization. Platonic friendships are almost automatically referred to possible boyfriend–girlfriend status. Jealousy brews in elementary school and junior high toward the girl who get the most attention from boys. The girls who ignore the calls to become sexualized are often seen as socially awkward or underdeveloped, or are socially shunned by their friends who have moved on.

Not long ago, I spoke with a mom whose family had recently relocated from a small town on the East Coast to the San Francisco Bay Area. Until the seventh grade, her daughter Dani had loved school and had been a good student. Dani was petite and lithe, with porcelain blue eyes and straight long brown hair. She was kind and sweet, and it was easy to see how she could be well liked. The problem that developed in the seventh grade, according to Dani's mother and some of her teachers, was that the boys started paying more attention to her. The other girls quickly became mean and spiteful. They called her a slut, and one of the most aggressive girls loudly accused Dani of sleeping with an eighth grade boy who was her friend. The boy in question came to Dani's defense, but the incident was just one of many demoralizing events that made up her seventh grade year. It is understandable that these social challenges had a marked impact on her academic experience and performance. She went from getting mostly A's to finishing the year with B's and C's. In one of our meetings, she readily exclaimed that the thing she wanted most was "a really good, true friend." She spent most of her eighth grade year participating in out-of-school activities in attempts to find other avenues for building friendships, and then attended a private high school without many of her junior high classmates.

Reason 3: Technology

IT'S EVERYWHERE AND ITS EFFECTS ARE EVERLASTING

Twenty or thirty years ago, students could potentially spend hours upon hours collecting research for a term paper. Researching often involved delving deep into a school's library stacks and spending hours looking at microfiche and photocopying important research papers from collective journals of the subject you were studying or the "annals of something important." When I was a junior in high school, I remember spending an entire Saturday afternoon at the local university library trying to track down literary research for my big honors English paper. Not only did I have to drive down to the University library but I also had to go through the lower-level stacks, find the right volume, make sure I had money on the copy card (remember those?), and hope that the copy machine was in order. Today, a well-informed student can do the same research that once took a half a day in a matter of minutes. Technology has utterly transformed the way in which we collect, digest, process, and comprehend information.

In schools, teachers and administrators are still tinkering with bringing technology into the classroom, and there is by no means one set standard. Some schools have gone to a one-to-one laptop or tablet system. Some students no longer carry around textbooks and are required to turn in their homework assignments by email (rather than hand in hard copy). Other schools are still trying to find the right online homework management system (which allows homework assignments and grades to be put online for parents and students to access); one school of nearly two thousand students near my office has gone through three different software systems over the past five years. Each adaptation has a ramp-up time to get all students and teachers onboard, and everyone involved must serially adapt to the ever-changing adaptations. Just when one system seems to work, it is replaced by something newer, faster, and supposedly better.

All this influx of technology has truly changed the way all our students are learning. No longer is it necessary to graph certain functions by hand because the graphing calculator will do it for us. Our calculators and our computers now serve as secondary and tertiary brains, and learning no longer consists of memorizing information that is now easily accessible, and there is an opportunity to move beyond regurgitating information to processing and applying information to come up with new solutions.

At the same time, the short-circuiting of process radically intensifies the easy access to vast digital storehouses. It requires only a little thought for students to hunt down ready-made answers to their questions. It takes only a few clicks on a search engine like Google to find a strong thesis statement for an essay on *Pride & Prejudice* or prefab assistance on any other conceivable topic. When all the reward is in the other direction—in passivity, in flawless regurgitating—girls can start to see the rational path for success to be simply following directions and doing exactly as they are told.

STUDENTS AND SOCIAL MEDIA

As a part of my work in schools, I often give interactive presentations to students on developing organization and time-management skills, setting goals, and finding a sense of personal purpose. One fall, I was invited to an American school abroad to talk to faculty, staff, and students. Many of the students at the school had moved at least once in the past five years due to their parents' jobs, often across countries or continents. Social networking was a vital tool for keeping them connected to their friends who were scattered around the globe. At the same time, the school faculty admitted that the junior high students, who had all recently received computers as part of the school's one-to-one laptop program, were struggling to juggle the demands of schoolwork with the temptation of digital socializing.

But even so, I was a little shocked when I asked how many of the hundred or so eleven-year-old sixth graders had Facebook accounts. When I then asked how many of the students used Facebook on a daily basis, virtually all of the hands shot up—even though Facebook had a rule at the time that users had to be above thirteen years old. Honestly, I shouldn't have been that surprised. In 2010, the Kaiser Family Foundation released their research findings in a report titled "Generation M²: Media in the Lives of 8- to 18-Year-Olds." Some of the study's findings were that nearly 40 percent of young people visit a social networking site on a typical day and that those who visit a social networking site spend nearly an hour there each day.[15]

In the last decade, digital social networking has exploded. At the time of this writing, the most recent available Nielsen study states that the average thirteen- to seventeen-year-old sends and receives over a hundred text messages each day. Female teenagers handle more texts than anyone: over four thousand each month, fully 60 percent more than their male counterparts, who are next on the list.[16] The many new social networking methods have increased in range and diversity, with multiple levels and layers of communication. A Facebook message can be responded to with a text, and a post on someone's Facebook wall can be a virtual RSVP for an event or a thank-you for a past invitation. The *social* is now virtually ever present. As a result, girls are not only predisposed to be interactive (as inherently group-oriented beings) but also are now almost literally plugged into the social forces, to the extent that it can be very difficult to turn their attention anywhere else. Home is no longer a safe haven from social pressure as girls constantly work to create and refine both their online and real-life images.

This is ever so true for members of our youngest generation, who have grown up with the Internet for their entire lives. I do not, of course, want to discount the many positive impacts of technological innovations. But school-age girls, who are in the process of learning to be more socially savvy than anyone else on the planet, are, by virtue of their saturation in the medium, perhaps most at risk from its abuses.

Four thousand text messages a month is a reflection of the fact that there are opportunities for girls to be social twenty-four hours a day, seven days a week. And this is crucial: It also means there is a correspondingly huge increase in the number of acts of being conditioned, shaped, and stamped by other people's thoughts. A young girl can post a photo of herself on Facebook wearing a new dress and receive instant feedback. A teenager can tweet a question and have any number of followers reply within minutes. If hypersexualization is learning to see oneself as disproportionately a sexual being, then there's a kind of corresponding hypersocialization, in which girls' media-driven social lives occupy an ever-larger proportion of their whole lives. It is not uncommon for girls (and yes, I know for more than a few adults as well) to sleep with their cell phones next to their pillows or for texting to be going on at two a.m. on a school night, well after the lights are supposed to be out.

These new technological challenges can be detrimental to the long-term social and emotional development of our girls, and we are just now starting to grasp the full extent of the effects. Every social move is now under a microscope. Indeed, the "Generation M²" report also noted that children now spend *over seven hours a day* on different entertainment media. In many cases, these kids end up media multitasking with different technological devices—texting while watching television, for example, or listening to music while surfing the Internet and chatting online with friends—so that they pack over ten hours of content into those seven hours of media time.[17] As a result, the price of a mistake is larger than in the past—and it's hard to develop healthy social habits when every possible mistake has such a huge audience and huge consequence. A 2012 study by Stanford University professor Cliff Nass concluded that young girls between the ages of eight and twelve years who most frequently shift across different technological devices and online systems (such as sending online messages, watching videos, or surfing the web) were the least likely to develop healthy social and emotional habits. To develop normal social behaviors, the study suggests that tween girls need to spend time communicating and interacting with friends and family face-to-face. Makes reasonable sense, except that it is happening less and less—among children *and* adults.[18] Indeed, the very nature of a digital medium like texting encourages more shallow relationships because individuals can manipulate what they want to text more than they could in a face-to-face conversation. Digital communication does not always lend itself to the deep, thoughtful, spontaneous conversations that can be pivotal to our young people's social and intellectual growth and development.

I am the first to admit that it is not easy to resist the temptations and excitement of technological advance and am in no way saying that technology is completely a bad thing—like most things, it's complicated. And even if we do see the drawbacks, it's hard to know what to do about it.

I've seen entire families eating out at a restaurant and each person using his or her phone or tablet—a new type of alone, together phenomenon. I know parents whose household rule that their middle school children use the Internet only in the living room has been thwarted by Internet-enabled smartphones. There are certainly ways in which parents can and should remain vigilant, but it can seem daunting and exhausting, especially for those who are not very technologically savvy. Just when you think you are up on the latest devices, something new comes along and explodes your carefully worked containment. As a result, most parents and educators are starting to realize that children need to learn how to self-regulate their use of technology, which is unfortunately easier said than done.

Indeed, students today are sent enormous mixed messages with technology—they need to use technology to be academically successful; however, that same technology can provide their greatest distraction from attaining academic success and personal fulfillment. According to the "Generation M^2" report, "About half of young people say they use media either 'most' (31%) or 'some' (25%) of the time they're doing their homework."[19] Indeed, one of the main reasons girls come to my office is because they struggle to manage their time and feel exhausted and overwhelmed. In part, this is owing to the need to be "on" all the time, which in turn drives the intense urge to multitask. Some girls try to convince me that they spend three to six hours on their homework every night, not even counting additional time for tests and projects. But when we walk through it in detail, step-by-step, it turns out that six hours of homework often means two hours of work fitted around four hours of low-level chatter of tweets, messages, and ten-second wall postings. For the typical teenager, quick and innocent texting adds up to over an hour and a half a day of sending and receiving messages.[20]

And beyond the time-management issues, there are some problems inherent to the medium. First and foremost, digital communication can create a false sense of intimacy for girls who are just starting to build their emotional and social resiliency. A classic case is a girl who feels connected to someone whom she has very little interaction with or has perhaps never even met IRL (in real life). Many of the junior high girls I work with tell of classmates who will regularly chat them up online but then ignore them at school. The shift to a digital communication style can cause simple misunderstandings, varying from "What did that text message really mean?" to "Why didn't she include me on that email list?" Even more detrimental, girls can feel more open to be uninhibitedly mean behind the hidden veil of the computer screen in a way that wouldn't be as likely in face-to-face interaction (not to say girls aren't mean to one another in person, because eye-rolling and snide contempt are still quite prevalent in school hallways and cafeterias across America).

In preparation for writing this book, I visited several junior high schools and high schools and met with girls from diverse backgrounds. We had collaborative, interactive, and fun discussions (there was a good bit of laughter involved). Consistently, the use of Formspring came up. Though not every girl had used the site, many had heard of some dramatic outcome from someone else's online experience. Formspring is a social networking site that allows users, without revealing their identities, to post questions and comments on others people's pages; the goal is to make it easier to break the ice and learn about others. Founded in 2009, Formspring boasts tens of millions of users and over four billion wall postings in its short existence.[21] The girls I met with used it as a way of posing questions that they were too scared to ask in person or to post statements on other people's profiles that they might never have said if they weren't anonymous. For junior high students, it can be a more technologically advanced way to ask, "Who do you like?"

Even if the intended purpose is to promote authentic openness, it was clear among the girls I talked with that using Formspring or other similar services can and does take a mean turn. One girl admitted that she would routinely find messages posted on her wall that said the world would be better off without her. She deleted the messages, and tried to act nonchalant when she shared the story, but it was easy to see that she was shaken. (She later shared that she had seen a therapist for past suicidal thoughts, but she didn't seem to link the anonymous posts to her own mental health challenges.) People tend to remember negative comments more than positive ones, and this can be ever so true for hypersensitive teenage girls. Formspring has a clear antibullying message on its website, and of course the vast majority of posts are benign. But the very existence of something like Formspring is in itself evidence that the Internet can directly encourage such styles of out-of-character and sometimes extreme behaviors. False voices that are disconnected from even a name may drown out genuine voices from real life. Indeed, huge swaths of the Internet are built entirely on the premise that people can act online as they never would elsewhere.

> The most insidious effect of technology's creep may be the disturbing reality that there's no time for reflection.

Finally, and perhaps most menacing, digital social interaction often drowns out other influences, including our own voices as we try to decide what we really want out of life. I think this is a largely unexamined factor in the feeling of many contemporary girls. After all, it's hard for girls to figure out who they really are and what they really like when they are being continually bombarded with messages, tweets, pokes, and prods that can keep them from ever having even one complete thought. The most insidious effect of technology's creep may be the disturbing reality that there's no time for reflection.

Reason 4: Differing Views of Healthy

Several times over the past few years I have visited students at 4C—the Adolescent Comprehensive Care Unit that is part of a hospital located about a mile from my office. It's a place that seems bright and cheery enough, though it is actually a locked-down facility where girls and boys stay when they are struggling with issues such as eating disorders and compulsive exercise addiction.

The past few times I have been there, I've visited girls who, after a routine physical examination, were found to have an incredibly low heart rate—so low, that doctors told them that they were at risk for a heart attack and immediately admitted them to the hospital. These were vibrant, active girls who ran and participated in varsity athletics and were seemingly well adjusted. Their peers would likely have described them as naturally slender or athletic looking. Each girl had started a massive exercise routine, running long distances and working out up to four hours a day and had not adjusted their eating habits accordingly. They were burning in excess of three or four thousand calories a day, and eating less than fifteen hundred calories, all while being clinically underweight. As a result, they were in fact so sick that they each had to go on complete bedrest (some for several months) to get back on the road to recovery.

For many girls, the conflicting stories about health contribute to a kind of routinely accepted but wholly abstract notion of improbable perfection—of a diffuse, elusive goal that can always be chased around one more bend. The focus is on external looks rather than internal health, and the result is often the emptiness that comes from never feeling good enough. There is always some new fitness program promising unprecedented results, some new eating advice; and with each comes the promise of eternal youth, toned abs, and firm butts. Indoor tanning has become a commonplace practice for girls seeking a "healthy" glow despite the stark truth that people who begin tanning before age thirty-five have a 75 percent higher risk of developing potentially fatal melanoma.[22] In the last decade alone, we've had so many different diet plans (often conflicting) touted by celebrities and self-proclaimed experts that it is difficult for a young person to discern fact from fiction. Girls as young as eight or nine announce that they are dieting, with very little understanding of what it authentically means to be healthy. Some girls going through puberty will reject their changing bodies by barely eating. As a result, many girls and young women develop troubling relationships with food early on.

We seem to be in a sort of warfare when it comes to the mental and physical health of girls today. More and more girls look healthy externally but are running on empty internally. Some follow nutritionally dubious diets filled with sugar, caffeine, and other quick-fix enablers that are profoundly detrimental to their long-term physical and emotional health. Other girls are so stressed out they use alcohol, prescription drugs or other narcotics, and/or self-mutilation (cutting) to cope with the intense pain and pressure from trying to meet and exceed so many never-ending external expectations. High-level club sports, with hours of practice and long weekends spent on high-intensity tournaments, are sometimes no longer functional exercise. Instead, the intense strain put on developing girls' bodies produces high rates of injuries that could potentially have long-term ramifications well into their adult lives.

A few years ago, a recent college graduate came to work in our office. She was tall, lean, and striking, with flowing blond hair and a clear complexion and looked to be a model of good health. But looks were deceiving in this case. She was working in our office for a few months before pursuing a medical degree, and her hyperintense ways left even the most energetic of us gasping for air. It soon became apparent that she subsisted on a regime of diet colas, intense exercise, super-caffeinated drinks, and mini snack packs of processed food and candies. She loudly opined about her extreme dislike of vegetables and ate fruits only rarely. It wasn't surprising to learn that she suffered from regular headaches and experienced dramatic mood swings. It *was* perhaps surprising that this future physician had yet to make the food–fuel connection, but in this way she was just like many of the girls I see, who are kept in the dark by the mixed messages of what is and isn't healthy.

What gets lost in this quest to look and be a certain way is the basic premise that each girl's body may be different in how it looks on the outside but similar in terms of a need to be supported with a nutritionally healthful diet.

THE CASE OF SLEEP DEPRIVATION

One telling effect of this hyperactive mentality is the almost epidemic proportions of sleep deprivation. Most parents nod vigorously when I talk about sleep in my presentations, but very few know the extreme depths of their children's deficits in this area. I often ask the parents how many of them know that their children have fallen asleep in class. Typically around 10 to 15 percent of parents raise their hands. When I ask the same thing of the students, nearly *every* hand is raised, even in the younger grades.

In talking with students, I am always amazed at how many students get less than seven hours of sleep per night; many function on as little as five or six. The older students get, the less they sleep; by twelfth grade, fully 72 percent of kids report sleeping less each night than they know they should to function at their best.[23] Research from the Centers for Disease Control and Prevention (CDC) reveals that 70.9 percent of girls get less than eight hours of sleep on an average school night.[24] Some of these girls are playing sports at a highly competitive level and managing a rigorous academic course load and extracurricular schedule; yet they are walking around in a near-catatonic state. The negative effects of sleep deprivation are well documented—crankiness, irritability, poor concentration, poor memory, immune deficiencies, anxiety, depression, lower academic achievement, and so on. Keep in mind that in war, sleep deprivation has often been used as torture, which is actually a good metaphor for the sad paradox of self-assault in the schools: The kids who are pushing themselves to do better at all costs are doing the very thing that will sabotage their ability to succeed.

In my student workshops and school presentations, I often do a simple math problem on sleep deprivation. The National Sleep Foundation suggests teenagers need somewhere between eight and a half and nine and a quarter hours of sleep per night (when I give these presentations, most of the students become temporarily fixated on the fact that there is a National Sleep Foundation).[25] I explain that by getting six hours of sleep, they are running a sleep deficit of at least two and a half hours every night, or twelve and a half hours per week. The students often nod knowingly as I multiply twelve and a half hours by thirty-five, the average number of weeks in a school year. It comes to over *forty* missed nights of sleep each year. Ears perk up, eyes widen. Most students are eager to do better in school. One simple way of doing so would be to step back, ease off the throttle, and get more sleep. While I do understand the difficulty of changing bad habits and going against the stream of extreme expectations, this is a battle worth fighting. The long-term mental and physical consequences far outweigh any benefits from striving to reach one more sleep-deprived accomplishment.

Reason 5: The Ultimate Myth

YOU CAN AND SHOULD HAVE IT ALL, ALL THE TIME

In the past, books on adolescent girls such as Mary Pipher's classic *Reviving Ophelia* focused on how girls can essentially shut down over the course of adolescence. The argument used to be that a cluster of natural and artificial influences was holding girls back; that, beginning in the sixth grade, girls were less likely to raise their hands or volunteer information in class, more apt to lose confidence in their abilities in math and science, and more likely to focus on their self-designated imperfections because of societal pressures. In the last few years, many of these assumptions have been revised, and many of the effects we used to think were societal are at least partially driven by stereotypes. Today, efforts have been made to redress these imbalances by empowering girls and young women to be leaders, encouraging them to drive fearlessly toward their goals, to refuse to take no for an answer, and not to back down. The notion of *girl power* has been drummed home, to the point that it can be credited in part with the scope of girls' current success. A 2012 Pew Research study revealed "young women [ages 18–34] now surpass young men in the importance they place on having a high-paying career or profession."[26] At the same time, a high percentage of young women think that marriage and family life are of great importance as well—giving the impression that more and more young women are increasingly determined to have it all—or to think they should want it all.

As I have said, girls are much freer, even in just the past two decades, to pursue different possibilities in ways that weren't as readily available in past generations. There have also been remarkable shifts in choices and opportunities that women are free to make with respect to the work and family ambitions. None of that, of course, in and of itself, is a bad thing. And certainly there remains work to be done. The math gap with boys is an important lingering area to remedy; as to some extent is the confidence gap. But overall it's almost as if the pendulum had swung too far in the other direction, and now *nothing is ever good enough.* Girls and young women are now bombarded with the message that they can and should be able to do it all, all the time. Now, not being successful at everything is akin to failure. This freedom to be all you can be develops into an unregulated pressure to be perfectly free and do it all, all the time—and it is no coincidence that today's girls are more anxious and struggle with greater rates of mental health issues than ever before. As one high school academic counselor from the Midwest explained to me, "These girls are so often expected to be finished products" rather than ever-evolving and changing young people. The girls I see feel as though they are constantly spinning around in circles. They need to be ambitious yet subdued, athletic yet feminine, intelligent yet flirty, and hardworking yet fun—the whole gamut of externally driven ideals.

> Now, not being successful at everything is akin to failure.

THE MYTH OF MULTITASKING

We hear the term *multitasking* all the time. Indeed, many schools are currently set up so that successful students often *have* to be great multi-taskers simply to encompass all the activities and workloads.

But here's the thing: None of us is truly good at multitasking. We want to believe that we are, and a lot of modern technological distractions count on us accepting it, but numerous studies show otherwise. In his book *Brain Rules*, John Medina notes, "the brain is a sequential processor, unable to pay attention to two things at the same time. Businesses and schools praise multitasking, but research clearly shows that it reduces productivity and increases mistakes."[27] The brain switches between the two (or more) things at hand, and nothing is accomplished with the same ability or depth that it would be if only one thing was mindfully focused on. When I talk to girls about listening to their favorite lyrical music while trying to write a paper, they readily admit that doing both at once simply doesn't work as much as they would like it to. One girl admitted to unwittingly writing the lyrics to the song down somewhere in the middle of a paragraph in her research paper, and only realizing it a few lines later.

A much more pervasive problem is the assumption—virtually built into students' overscheduling—that doing multiple things at once is something we *want* to be good at. Rather than putting the emphasis on concentration, focus, and attention and clearing girls' schedules to promote these skills, we praise them for piling on more and more. Most students will brag about their multitasking prowess as a skill, when in actuality it undermines their performance and makes them feel less satisfied and more stressed.

The Perfect Girl Problem

For some girls, *effortless perfection* describes how they think they are supposed to be able to do everything flawlessly with little or no perceived effort and gives them an ideal to hide behind when things start to spiral out of control. For some, it conjures up the image of how they are supposed to show up to school looking fresh-faced and dewy, with perfect hair and makeup, and float through school, acing tests with little preparation and maintaining an active social life. Even though that effortlessly perfect girl exists with about as much frequency as unicorns in the forest, the myth of effortless perfection leads many girls to feel less worthy when they believe they don't meet up to the unobtainable standards and causes them to be more likely to hide their problems rather than seek solutions.

In today's world, too many girls believe that being perfect (however *perfect* is defined in their world) is an idealized standard to strive toward. As a result, they grapple with issues that fester and become larger and more intense than they need to (wonder what a girl is doing in her bedroom for hours? Think she is focused on homework? Maybe. But she might well be overanalyzing the troubles she perceives to be accumulating in her life). In a world of unobtainable perfection, being vulnerable is seen as being weak, and needing help is reduced to being needy. Instead of dealing with problems and actively seeking solutions, many girls turn to avoidance, hiding, and compensatory behaviors to mask the underlying anxiety and fear they experience from not fully confronting their challenges.

Leaning Forward, Falling Backward, Getting It Right

I want to end the chapter by thinking through some of the temptations of the achievement culture. So much of the success that girls are striving to achieve is actually fake success or empty success: It is based on the box-filling model of internalizing someone else's wishes (academic, sexual, appearance-obsessed, or technologically reverberated), and then treating oneself like the object of those wishes. The appeal of the proverbial Gold Star—getting outward praise and external accolades—can be too powerful an elixir to overcome. The temptations of achievement obsession are everywhere, and it is extraordinarily difficult to change direction or even to identify the need to do so, especially when everyone and everything is telling you to keep pushing forward. So many young women I have talked with in their middle to late twenties have realized, after spending an inordinate amount of time and money on college and graduate school, that they feel stuck in a career path they do not care about. Almost universally, they wish someone had encouraged them to reflect on their interests and develop their own sense of personal purpose earlier in their lives. Instead, they were swept along by the mass, unquestioning consensus to achieve more, accomplish bigger, and spend time accumulating, all at the expense of building a vision of personal satisfaction. In a well-circulated *Forbes* article aptly titled "Why Millennial Women Are Burning Out at Work by 30," one young woman surmised that the burnout happens because "they [young women] don't know what they are striving for, which makes it really hard to move forward."[28]

Why are you pursuing that job? What finish line are you racing toward? Is all the sacrifice worth it? The only way these inevitable questions can ultimately lead a woman *forward* into more intense, engaging, successful work is if she has taken the time and effort, probably as a girl in school, to develop self-awareness and figure out the shape of her own personal sense of purpose.

Though it certainly may seem that girls today face an uphill battle in the quest to find personal, social, and academic fulfillment, it's important to recognize that we can make a difference if we encourage girls to reflect carefully about what they really want in their world. In the upcoming chapters, I explore the many incremental and meaningful ways we can offer support by collaborating with our girls to find significant solutions. I have included corresponding exercises to serve as suggestions and conversation starters. The exercises help provide a framework of understanding and a toolbox of ideas to start from, though I recognize that what works for one girl may not work for another. The strategies can and should be adapted and individualized to work within the context of what is right for your parent–daughter dynamic. And perhaps you aren't the right one to approach some of the topics, and another person's efforts would elicit a more favorable response. Maybe an aunt or family friend or mentor would be a better person, or someone else altogether. (Indeed, that is why so many students find their way to my office.) Regardless, we need to work with our girls earlier, as part of their standard development and education, to become more conscious of their choices, of the powers of their own choice, both for and against what they and others desire. At the same time, teaching girls to develop empathy and compassion for themselves, as well as for others, allows them to look inward to reflect on their own dreams, desires, and interests and begin to fill the emptiness that has become so pervasive among our girls and young women.

||||||||||||||||||||

CHAPTER TWO

So Many Ways to Be Boxed In

When Susan first called our office about her daughter Rebecca, her concern came through the phone line loud and clear. As she explained when we spoke, Rebecca's grades had plummeted in her first semester of seventh grade. Some of the problem was obviously organizational—now in middle school, Rebecca was juggling six different classes with different teachers who had different sets of expectations, rather than just the one classroom teacher whose preferences she knew and felt comfortable with. She also certainly struggled with time management: Her mom reported that she could spend hours staring at the wall in her room or messaging with friends under the guise of completing her homework (I provide more suggestions on organization and time management in Chapters 5 and 6). As I went on to meet and work with Rebecca, it became apparent that a much greater problem was her changing social world. She had just gone from a small elementary school to a much bigger middle school, where she was one of many more students vying to find and maintain friendships, trying to figure out the hierarchies, and struggling to navigate the lunchtime scene—all while needing to get to class on time and to complete her homework with some semblance of understanding.

It was a lot for anyone to juggle, let alone a preteen going through puberty. It was obvious that the mental and emotional energy Rebecca was expending on social survival was leaving her drained and distracted in the classroom. In the last fifteen minutes of one of her morning classes, Rebecca was frequently caught up in her own world, thinking about where she would sit at lunch, who would be there, and which boy she might talk to. As a result, she would forget to record the day's homework. Similar small lapses were happening all over her schedule, and they were adding up to a serious problem. Both Rebecca and her mother were frustrated by the situation, and Rebecca's mom was perplexed about how to help.

Socially, school can be tough for girls, no matter where they are on the social spectrum. As girls move through junior high and high school, there are a million cues to take in and interpret—about preferred and proscribed behaviors, about social hierarchies and cliques, about whom to like, and how to be—as I discuss in this chapter, so many ways to be boxed in. As in many of the facets of student life I will be describing, the calls to conform to acceptable norms have gotten louder, even as the norms themselves have become much more tightly defined. Alexandra Robbins, in *The Geeks Shall Inherit the Earth*, argues that such a narrowing of norms is one of the reasons "that student bullying is up, self-esteem is down, and social warfare is fierce."[1]

As most parents with both sons and daughters can attest to, girls tend to internalize social information and then analyze what they internalize much more than their male peers. This is a basic, though obviously not universal, difference in developmental and learning styles that in part guides my different practices with girls and boys.[2] Whereas the boys who come into my office tend to struggle with the nuts and bolts of organization and time management (for example, Did you turn in that assignment? Where is the soccer uniform you were supposed to return two weeks ago?), girls often struggle with the intersection of the social and academic sides of school—in particular with learning to value their own sense of self and their gifts and abilities within a sea of cultural expectations. Once given a system to follow, girls adopt it faster; think about the girls who obsessively color coordinate their notebooks, who rotate five different highlighter colors, or who alphabetize their flashcards. The bigger challenge for girls is that they run the risk of becoming *too* self-organizing, too self-accommodating, too externally well matched to school demands at the risk of neglecting other, important internal aspects of themselves.

Some of the girls I work with admitted to coming up with organizational systems that were so complex and complicated they weren't able to keep up easily with all their self-imposed regulations. Girls can overcompensate in attempts to find a system that will be the answer to all their social and emotional struggles that impact the academic ones. Other girls who struggle academically simply check out and shift their efforts elsewhere because they feel there is far too much to do and they don't know where to start. School administrators repeatedly tell me that girls are all too good at hiding from rather than addressing the issues that bother them, and that the problem often lurks just below the surface.

In this chapter, I present a portrait gallery of girls in school, as they are today, as I see them day by day. I present these pictures in the form of different socioeducational styles; I want to capture what is typical in girls' way of navigating the box-filling, self-emptying demands I have described in the previous chapter. The character profiles are composites of actual students I have worked with but in no way am I suggesting that every Socially Centered Starlet is sexually promiscuous or that every Worst-Case Scenario Worrier is likely to attempt suicide. What I am suggesting, though, is that beneath the surface of everyday life for many girls exists a darkness and pain that results from box-filling behavior and its ensuing emptiness. Many parents and educators will recognize girls they know in one or several of these composite pictures. Chances are, one or more of these socioeducational styles resonates with

haps the girl you have in mind is a bit of a Caring Considerate
er with a smidgen of Worst-Case Worrier and is at risk of
turning into an Overstressed Overachiever. You may even see yourself.
I've developed these snapshots for just that reason: to help readers start
thinking about finding personalized solutions for the girls and young
women in their lives.

The Overstressed Overachiever

Kate has never met a mountain she hasn't wanted to climb—literally
and figuratively. She takes an academically rigorous course load and is
intensely involved with many activities both in and outside of school.
She runs cross-country and track, and volunteers at the children's hospital near her home. She is diligent and conscientious, and will often go
to school when sick to avoid missing a crucial class or activity. Most
nights she is up late perfecting an assignment, organizing a group project for school, or baking a cake for her friend's birthday. She is involved
in everything, all the time and will often keep going at top speed until
she is mentally and physically exhausted. At that point, she typically
has a mini-breakdown characterized by crying and yelling, withdraws
into her cocoon to recuperate, reemerges full of new energy, and then
starts the cycle all over again. A few years ago, she took up running as
a healthy stress-reliever, but now she has begun to take that to extremes
as well, going on longer and longer runs in the name of relaxation. She
has suffered from shin splints and a stress fracture and spent several
months last year in an orthopedic boot after she ignored her doctor's
initial warnings because she loves the endorphin high and gets grumpy
when people tell her to take a break.

Kate is hyperorganized, to the point of often creating extra work for
herself. She is a list maker, a doer, and a girl who achieves at breakneck
speed. Her academic and extracurricular résumé is long and detailed,

and her calendar is sometimes double- and triple-booked. She feels antsy when she has nothing to do, has few if any hobbies, and would feel disoriented and anxious at the idea of spending the day free from obligations. She stays up late and gets up early with such regularity that it is rare for her to function without some sort of caffeine or sugar fix to get her through the day.

Kate is a spinning top, sometimes zipping along to superior numbers achievement, sometimes grindingly overwhelmed, alternating between going a hundred miles an hour and wobbling to a complete stop. To the outside world, she is a constant success, because her collapses are hidden from all but her parents and closest friends. She is proud and fierce, and to her peers, someone who magically "does it all."

Kate is diligent, motivated, and seemingly self-directed. She is often extremely achievement-oriented and can seem like a dream child or student, except when she is in the midst of a meltdown. In taking everything to the highest level possible, she struggles to distinguish *sufficient* from *excessive*. Because she equates doing more with success, she thinks *relaxation* means "failure." In the past decade, I have seen more and more Overstressed Overachiever girls in my office. Their bursting planners make it easy to identify their constant pervading fear that they are not doing enough. Of course there is nothing wrong with hopes, dreams, and ambition. But the underlying fragility, which stems directly from their hyperactive box filling, makes them likely to come to a point at which they just might snap.

My usual first step with a student like Kate is to take a look at her schedule and identify precisely how she is spending her time. We use the Weekly Flow Chart (page 100) to map out her time commitments in a detailed, fine-grained way. We also talk about other important factors in day-to-day self-management and wellness: crucially, food as a fuel source and sleep as the bedrock of health, learning, and overall wellness. Sometimes, this can be a back and forth process before we make any real progress; she is scared of giving something up and ends up piling more and more things into the empty spaces we've cleared. Eventually, we try to incorporate hobbies in hopes that she can cultivate her own sense of personal enjoyment and fun.

The Socially Centered Starlet

Alissa is bubbly, effusive, and energetic; it's hard not to notice her cheery disposition when she walks into a room. It's not surprising that she has a reliable group of friends who are drawn to her effervescence. A solid-B student, she spends her weekends playing volleyball and bouncing between her friends' houses for sleepovers, school projects, and hanging out. She is a garrulous multitasker, constantly chatting with someone, either in real life (IRL) or online, about the latest and greatest news or gossip. She may not seem to care as much about the academic side of school (though she does), but she has the social piece down. Her emotional intelligence is high, and she manages to spend a disproportionate amount of her time in the school halls soaking up information about everything and everyone. Her clothes and makeup highlight her position at the center of attention.

Though Alissa is a great communicator, she often fears she is missing out and worries that something crucial will be happening in the few moments that she is not in touch—and in this new age of texting and handheld technology, she can be almost constantly tapped in. Her phone often goes to bed with her; it is the last thing she checks before going to sleep and the first thing she checks in the morning. Her parents tried to limit her phone usage, but basically gave in as they felt it wasn't a battle worth fighting or that they could possibly win. Alissa easily sends over two hundred text messages a day, and routinely juggles four or five conversations at once. She sits with her lunch group while tapping out messages on her phone to those down the hall or at a neighboring school. Her weekdays are spent making plans for the weekend, and she feels genuine stress when social plans don't turn out as expected or she has tension with one of her friends.

Alissa believes that her social life is the most important part of her existence. She thrives on being in the vortex of her school's social scene, where the currents of information and influence are strongest. But her drive to maintain popularity often comes at a cost, and she struggles with developing her own self-awareness in the midst of trying to achieve social success. On weekends, her hard partying ways can be the fodder of Monday morning stories: She is the fun-time girl whose alcohol-fueled craziness and late-night activities are the ways that she lets loose and compensates for her underlying hum of social anxiety and pressure. Her primary challenge is to be more than merely absorptive of other people's thoughts and moods; she needs to figure out what she really wants, beyond the whirlwind, rather than constantly being a people-pleaser.

Socially Centered Starlets like Alissa typically need to reflect on how they are spending time—whether it is all just being tossed around in the storm of relationships, news, and plans for the weekend. It is often helpful for them, for the goal of getting their feet back on the ground, to specifically identify ways to reverse their usual patterns—for example, to give to others rather than simply feeding off the social scene, and to figure out what their own interests are separate from their technological overload. Learning organizational and time-management strategies was crucial for forcing Alissa to distinguish, right there on the paper, between academic and social pursuits and gave her the chance to focus on one or the other without having to juggle several pieces at once. Having required breaks from technology, by creating a Technology Box and enforcing Technology Curfews (discussed in Chapters 5 and 6), provided a period of calm. Finding ways to decompress and learn what stillness and silence feel like can be critical to a Socially Centered Starlet's overall emotional and social development. More important, it can be part of the longer-term plan to ensure that Alissa makes time to be alone and gets used to it, away from the whirl of other people she typically depends on for short-term sustenance.

The Pensively Private Thinker

Most teachers would describe Marie as quiet and shy, though her written work reveals a young woman with complex creative thoughts and interests. Ever since elementary school, Marie has spent the majority of her weekday afternoons and weekends at the local dance school by her house. She was a beautiful dancer until she was sidelined by a back injury the summer after her eighth grade year. Her disappointment from her inability to dance was compounded by her parents' stealth separation. Though she and her two siblings knew their mom was going to file for divorce, their father couldn't move out of the family home because of his recent unemployment. The family's financial strain was a source of pressure for Marie's parents, who did not talk openly about their situation. Regardless, Marie could sense the stress but felt as though she had no outlet; she hadn't let her friends know about her parents' impending divorce and felt embarrassment and shame about their financial situation, and her injury left her feeling as though she had no escape from the daily pressures of her school and family. After her mom discovered that Marie was cutting herself as a way to assuage the stress and pain she was feeling, Marie started seeing a therapist once a week. The therapist was friendly and reassuring, but even after ten sessions Marie had yet to even mention her parents' impending divorce.

Physically, Marie could be described as demure and plain, avoiding any fashions she regards as overly dramatic. In all sorts of ways, she plays it safe. She has always been a private person and an intense analyzer, but with adolescence she has become even more pensive and less collaborative, and often second-guesses herself and her decisions. In school, she is conscientious and reliable; her written work actually reveals a thoughtful expressiveness rarely on display in classroom discussions or activities. Among her peers, she is somewhat of an afterthought socially—she has a loosely defined group of friends whom she sits with at lunch and interacts with regularly, but they don't feel like they know her because she is not much of a sharer. Though she does communicate with friends online occasionally and responds to texts as they come in, as a Pensively Private Thinker, she is not likely to be proactive in making plans or developing relationships. Her friends sometimes forget to include her in social events because she is more of a fringe member of the group than a core contributor.

Outwardly, she usually seems unfazed by the social oversights because she is reluctant to express her feelings. Marie belongs to a few clubs but is reluctant to truly commit herself to new things or take risks for fear of how she might be perceived or judged. Part of her shyness owes not merely to a solitary nature, but to attaching *too* much credence to other people's opinions. As a result, she is never fully engaged, and can easily be sidetracked by comments and criticisms (constructive or otherwise) from friends, family, teachers, and other adults.

Marie has a lot going on inside her head, but not much of it is actively revealed until she is past the point of being overwhelmed. Her major challenges are learning confidence in expressing her thoughts and developing a more balanced communication style that doesn't swing so widely between silence and meltdown. Encouraging her written expression (via journaling or creative writing), where she feels safer, allows her to rehearse expressive modes and ultimately serves as a bridge into greater conversational ease. Her other challenge is learning how to identify and then to take healthy social and emotional risks. Finding a way to become an active member of a community where she feels accepted—either inside or outside of the school setting—can make her life feel much more engaged. Setting the goal of trying a new activity or academic endeavor or starting a conversation with a new classmate can show her how capable she is of being more connected to the various circles of her life.

The Caring Considerate Peacemaker

Mercedes was one of the most thoughtful, kind, and generous young women I had the opportunity to work with as a college adviser. Warm and bubbly, she always had something genuinely nice to say about everyone; her exuberance was infectious. Academically, she worked diligently to get her homework done and do well in school and was generally a conscientious student. In class, though she would participate, she would never stretch herself beyond benign answers to rudimentary questions. She avoided confrontational topics or saying anything that might seem controversial for fear of creating a dispute or argument. She lived with both parents and was the middle child; her older and younger sibling were both much more outgoing and opinionated. Mercedes seemed to work overtime to try to keep her life smooth and conflict-free. She remembered birthdays with cards and cakes and would readily go out of her way to invite someone who was sitting alone to join her at the lunch table. She would write an encouraging note to someone who was going through a rough time—her sensitivity knew no bounds.

She always wanted to do the right thing, and she prized and sought to create a sense of harmony that doesn't always exist in adolescent relationships. At the beginning of high school, she struggled to find a group of friends because she was a little more vulnerable socially; she didn't fit her peers' definition of *cool* or *hot* and lacked the edge of meanness and command that often breeds self-selective perceived popularity. As she made her way through high school, Mercedes learned how to develop friendships based on mutual understanding and how to address little disputes and challenges positively rather than avoiding them. By her senior year, most of her peers and teachers would agree that the world could use a few more young people like Mercedes.

Caring Considerate Peacemakers like Mercedes avoid conflict and prefer situations free of the drama and stress that pervade the lives of many teenage girls. They like being liked and love to help out whenever they can. But they can also be passive and won't fight to change their schedule to get the class they want or confront a friend who has been hurtful because they would rather go along with a situation that is less than ideal than create what they perceive would be major waves (which are more like minor ripples). As a result, however, they are vulnerable to being taken advantage of. These girls can sometimes be left holding the bag because they are loyal and will take the fall, and they can be treated poorly by those who are more socially sophisticated and aggressive.

Girls who have some of the qualities like Mercedes are among the loveliest young people to be around—in a world as crazy as ours can be, they give us hope for the future. They are healers and soothers; they take off some of the rough edges of modern life. But in order for that kindness to not be exploited, they need to learn confidence and that not all conflict is negative. Learning how to negotiate *within* conflict, and create win–win situations, is a natural extension of their gifts and will benefit everyone by spreading their influence over a wider sphere.

The Dramatic Queen of the Party

Socially dominant and aggressive, Brooke was a true Dramatic Queen of the Party. In an average lunch period, Brooke could manipulate friends and classmates with the easy know-how of a seasoned politician. She alternated between being funny, vibrant, and outrageous, all in the name of having a good time and being the center of attention. Most of her classmates would agree that Brooke had *perceived* popularity—that is, she is well known among her peers and fits the teenage definition of appeal, even though many of her classmates were privately fearful of her wrath. Her outfits were tight, low-cut, and slightly inappropriate, and she would occasionally serve after-school detentions for being out of the school dress code. Her makeup was just as dramatic as her personality, with a thick slab of black eyeliner framing her almond-shaped eyes and bright colors of intense eye shadow and blush completing the look.

Brooke focused her attention on the social aspects of her school day, drawing in the latest gossip and generating new story lines to fuel the fire that is the drama of teenage life. She could create mountain ranges of emotional tumult out of something as seemingly simple as who was sitting with whom at lunch, or who got a ride home with whom after practice. She lived for masterminding the weekend party scene and analyzing who would be riding in the car together to the Friday night football game. She didn't usually seem to care if someone got hurt as long as she and her friends were taken care of. But although her friends seemed a tight-knit group, the group's dynamics could turn on a dime. Brooke was in the middle of it all, stirring the pot and fanning the flames. She had no problem manipulating her friends and turning the group against one girl—and did so with such regularity that everyone was kept anxious and hyperaware.

Though boys thought she was attractive, Brooke had intense insecurities about her looks and was incredibly hard on herself about her appearance. She would routinely starve herself or try a variety of fad diets, and her alcohol consumption at parties would make her do things she would forget. She blacked out more than a few times; though her parents knew she drank, they had little indication of her significant level of alcohol consumption and the dangerous behaviors that followed. More than a few times, she had hooked up with a guy and not remembered the details afterward, and she regularly lied to her friends and her parents based on a convenient image she wanted to portray. More than once she had betrayed a friend in attempts to get a guy she had her eye on, which rotated with more frequency than she liked to admit. She usually told her parents she was sleeping over at someone's house, so they rarely saw her at the end of an evening.

It would be easy to describe Brooke as a mean girl or a Queen Bee, but the truth was much more complex. The academic side of school did not come as easily to her, and Brooke found the social piece to be more exciting. It's what she felt she was good at. She had a high level of emotional intelligence, which was not readily rewarded on quizzes and tests, though she could talk her way out of many situations with teachers who secretly feared her. Even at a very young age, Brooke was incredibly astute at analyzing complex interpersonal relationships and figuring out how to use such situations to her advantage. She was masterful at hiding her own emotional insecurities behind a veil of a hard-charging, somewhat promiscuous party girl who fed on the drama she created or contributed to.

Girls like Brooke are highly emotional, somewhat self-focused and self-involved girls who can be the life of the party and every teacher's worst nightmare. Many current reality shows are filled with one or more participants who have similar characteristics. Their underlying intentions are pretty much all about themselves and their needs. These girls can be aggressive socially and will call out in class with a clever comment that has an underlying meanness. They can silence their classmates with their brusque attitude and make others feel physically and mentally small. They are thrilled to be in the know and seem to love confrontation—all drama, all the time. But there is a particular fragility to their performances. Underneath the shiny exterior is often a confused internal mess. The emotionally charged situations they seek out are an exacerbation of their own precarious psychic state. Mentally and spiritually, girls like Brooke may struggle because they don't take the time to develop their personal potential, which is often quite high. They may find social comfort in the consistent use of alcohol and drugs as a way to maintain their party-girl image. And because they are so invested in their public persona, facing adversity or failure can cause an acutely uncomfortable disorientation.

For Dramatic Queens of the Party like Brooke, developing empathy skills is crucial. The key is to recognize and channel their enormous magnetism and personal energy. A situation in which they help others and develop their self-worth can be incredibly challenging to their normal outlook. But for just this reason, it can incite a level of self-reflection they have likely avoided in the past. Girls who have, for example, a completely novel experience in nature or of helping those in need, can learn to flip their aggressiveness into an intensity of meaningful engagement.

The Creative Wonder

Marianne came to see me at the beginning of her sophomore year because she was struggling in school, particularly in math. Every time she came into my office, she would have on a very fashion-forward outfit—not trendy but more following some private inspiration and certainly not in line with what the typical high school student was wearing. She was thoughtful and reflective, and we would have discussions about her most recent art piece or a literary work she had read in class that she found especially moving.

Often, though, Marianne would become stressed at the amount of academic schoolwork she had and was easily overwhelmed. She found it tough to manage all the demands of her competitive high school, largely due to her commitment to art, her favorite class, which absorbed most of her time. We worked on sharpening her organizational and time-management skills, which was not a foolproof solution but did ultimately reduce her stress by allowing her to streamline her schoolwork so she could focus on art, which naturally took an enormous amount of time and attention. She loved losing herself in a new project or piece—the immersion was part of the pleasure. Marianne could work for hours, without a set start and finish or any sense of what it meant to be done beyond her own aesthetic judgment, and for this she would receive no more official credit than for a long set of math problems, though for her the reward was immeasurably greater.

Her parents supported her passion but wondered why she couldn't at least submit her homework on time and do better on math tests. Though she had friends, the typical high school experience was not something that went along with her dreams.

Artistic, wondrous, and curious, Creative Wonders like Marianne are the epitome of what our system disallows. They can easily become lost in our current academic environment. Their artistic endeavors take a great deal of time and energy and rarely receive the same accolades as more cut-and-dried academic achievements. Often, as they get older, girls like Marianne are forced to make a choice either to abandon their artistic loves because they are too all-consuming or to alienate themselves from the academic setting because it's not flexible enough to grow with their sense of personal purpose.

Ironically, however, new technology has made our world ever more in need of the innovativeness and creativity; we need our girls to be fully engaged and in tune with their talents now more than ever. The real question is not how practical or impractical their interests are but how Creative Wonders can make the passage through school to the world waiting to receive them with their vision intact. Unfortunately, our academic and social structures often exclude girls like Marianne from an early age. Too often, they are sacrificed to the need to get on with more conventional kinds of success. Put simply, girls who have creative talents and interests should be encouraged to nurture their artistic skills alongside their academic ones. These are the rare girls who already know their core desires and interests. Finding ways to incorporate their talents within the framework of academic life is not only humane; it's part of the change in perspective, toward recognizing the central importance of individual purpose and vision, that we should adopt for all our girls.

The starting point for Marianne was the commitment to maintaining her artistic focus because it is genuine and deep. Pursuing artistic endeavors is not an expendable sideshow to her life; it is right at the heart of it. And even for girls whose commitment is not all-out, it is invariably in these cases an expression of real interest, which should be respected for its own sake. Marianne designed an independent study (her school allowed this) so her serious work could be given the space it needed to unfold. For some Creative Wonders, it might be better to block out one or two afternoons per week to focus on art projects (and yes, this can and should happen). Cultivating a community of like-minded friends and mentors—and helping these girls get in touch with such resources—can provide a niche for girls like Marianne, who are perhaps socially adrift or pressed by demands that do not always further their pursuit of their personal interests.

The Constant Chameleon

To see Amie in the different arenas of her life, one might think that she had multiple personalities. With her friends at school or in my office, she was energetic and engaging, full of sharp commentary and witty remarks. In the classroom, her behavior and performance varied according to the teacher's personality and teaching style. At home, she was quiet in response to the energy levels of her much older parents. On the soccer field, where she spent hours after school, she was a reliable, strong, and determined presence with her teammates and coach. She succeeded in all these environments in part due to her emotional intelligence, which made her wonderful at anticipating the needs of others and fitting in.

But her changeability was also a symptom of her struggle to figure out her own needs and interests, apart from those of other people she sought to please. If her friends wanted to go to the movies, she would go to the movies. If they wanted to hang out at the mall, she went to the mall. At some level, being easygoing and flexible, both wonderful qualities, had become a version of complacency. Over time, she exhausted herself tracking what everyone wanted from her; the many scenes and spheres of her life were too much to anticipate and manage and mix herself into. To assuage the pain, she started popping different types of pills—at first it was just a few Advil or Tylenol. Then she found the extra pain meds that her mom had left lying around from her knee surgery, and pretty soon, Amie was hooked on finding some way to take the edge off. By the time she turned eighteen, she had spent $75 to get a doctor to write a prescription for medicinal marijuana, which is legal in the state of California. Without her parents' knowledge, she had a stash of pot that she baked into brownies and shared with friends at school as their way of getting through the day.

More than anything, the Constant Chameleon blends in and blends in well. She avoids conflict at all costs, and her avoidance often comes at the high price of sacrificing her own identity. She takes on different roles with her friends and family and is influenced by whomever she is with at the moment. She gets along with pretty much everyone but has no distinctive characteristics or quirks, at least none that she allows to determine the relationships she's in. As a result, she can quickly get lost in the interests and expectations of others without developing her own. Though her adaptability and ability to understand her audience could serve her well later in life in a professional setting, she runs the risk of never developing an authentic voice inside and outside the classroom. She habitually bows to external pressure; she is, in effect, continually training herself to seek the box-filling approval of those around her.

When working with students like Amie, I frequently encourage them to comfortably be themselves outside their social adaptations. Developing an internal sense of self and resiliency to conflict is important, as is helping these girls explore and discover their own interests, opinions, and sense of purpose.

The Worst-Case Scenario Worrier

In high school, Jenn would sit in the front row of every classroom, with her hand often raised high while simultaneously taking frantic notes. She frequently overprepared for tests and quizzes; her razor-sharp focus on grades and results made her a good, though also a fairly mechanical, student. Though school did not come easy to her, her anxiety-fueled work ethic—bred from worry—was absolutely amazing. Sitting behind her in class, you could almost see the steam coming out of her ears as she bore down on her responsibilities. On Wednesdays and Thursdays, she trained the same dogged focus on the details of the upcoming weekend: Who was going in what car for the football game? What parties were going on? On group projects, her micromanaging annoyed her partners to no end, though they also knew Jenn's flood of worry would probably carry them to a top grade.

Jenn's worrisome ways also translated in her body image and perception of herself. Whenever she looked at herself in the mirror, she tormented herself with negative self-talk—her nose was too big, her chest too flat, and her thighs were huge. She would typically count calories with the same precision she paid to her schoolwork and punish herself when she thought that she was "bad" in relation to her eating habits. Disappointments would fuel an emotional eating spree, in which tortilla chips, brownies, guacamole, candy, cake, and pizza could be demolished in rapid succession until her stomach hurt. Sometimes, she would make herself throw up to try and curb her guilt. At the end of a particularly stressful week, she got caught in the lie of being at a party on a local college campus when she told her parents that she was going to spend the night at her friend's house. Her parents were furious, and she panicked, swallowing a bunch of pills. She ended up at the hospital emergency room, where her stomach was pumped. She attended several therapy sessions before she decided she didn't need it anymore, and her parents were more than willing to put it behind them as well. Jenn's parents had a hard time grasping the gravity of her behavior and preferred that as few people knew about their daughter's erratic behavior as possible. They wrote off her suicide attempt as an impulsive act born out of fear and not a signal of a greater problem.

Worst-Case Scenario Worriers like Jenn exhaust themselves by overthinking everything—academic, social, personal, extracurricular, and otherwise. They are anxious, and their anxiety is readily apparent to those around them. The idea of relaxing and letting go is uncomfortable in a skin-crawling sort of way. New situations are especially worrisome. They like routines and schedules, and thrive in number-wise academic environments that are structured and predictable. Academically, they worry about tests and quizzes and short- and long-term projects and cannot be dissuaded from giving small assignments much more effort than they require. Their perfectionist tendencies sometimes keep them from being able to judge when a project is finished (because there is always more that can be done!). Socially and emotionally, they are easily overwhelmed and need constant reassurance from others, though external encouragement is only a temporary panacea.

What girls who worry excessively really need to do is to slow down and figure out why they are worried so much of the time, which is generally not an easy task. Developing coping strategies or ways in which to redirect the energies of Worst-Case Scenario Worriers like Jenn can be particularly helpful and usually require active efforts and consistent reinforcement. Once such girls feel comfortable thinking directly about the nature of their anxiety, and whether it is serving their aims (which they usually have not articulated even to themselves), they are ready to think further, beyond worries, into the realm of personal satisfaction, fulfillment, and purpose.

This book is designed to help parents, educators, and girls themselves recognize and understand these common challenges and then to give them the tools to work their way back from box filling to a bedrock of personal purpose. In the chapters that follow, I offer an overarching plan filled with suggestions that cover time, space, organizational styles, social and emotional growth, study skills, and spiritual development. It's a big task, but then again, it's a big problem that many of our girls and young women are facing. So, take a deep breath, visualize positive changes, and let's begin.

||||||||||||||||||||||

CHAPTER THREE

Parental Attitudes and Approach

Part of the Problem or Part of the Solution?

Visionary computer legend and Apple founder Steve Jobs once said, "You can't connect the dots looking forward; you can only connect them looking backwards. So you have to trust that the dots will somehow connect in your future. . . . Because believing that the dots will connect down the road will give you the confidence to follow your heart even when it leads you off the well worn path; and that will make all the difference."[1] No one has any idea how his or her life is really going to turn out, and many of the most interesting people in the world rarely lead methodically linear lives. True geniuses and exceptionally successful people don't fear life because they refuse to constrict themselves by needing someone's validation for everything they do. When they try something that fails, it's not a judgment on their intrinsic worth.

One of the themes of this book is that adopting a more experimental, purposeful, and personally fulfilling outlook is a serious challenge for girls in today's culture. On every side they are pulled to conform to other people's standards; living through themselves for others, many girls *do* relate to their lives as though they were in fear. But this is a pattern of social development we can change. Ours is an extraordinarily demanding time, but it is also a time rich in innovation. New possibilities and opportunities open up daily that can potentially inspire girls to evolve, take risks, and grow.

Over the last few decades, the limits of our world have virtually exploded. In nearly every field of endeavor, there now exist whole new categories of opportunities. This plethora of possibilities, while it can be daunting, represents a great resource for parents and educators in their work to widen girls' views of what they can meaningfully do. There is enormous risk for girls to get lost in the superficialities of our culture, but given our consciousness of that fact, there is also great opportunity to break down the boxes of unhealthy habits of thought. My advice, if parents really want to embolden their daughters to think for themselves, is for them to embrace the opportunities found in new kinds of fulfilled lives, break down the boxes, and work to create a world outside the box.

Parents: Part of the Problem?

I recently had a mother and father come in for a parent consultation because they were worried about their daughter's lack of motivation, initiative, and tenacity. Their daughter, Campbell, was a high school junior and a solid-B student at an academically competitive school in the San Francisco Bay Area. She was engaged in activities she enjoyed and had some relatively close friends but really didn't love the high school social scene. She wasn't aggressive or overly competitive, though she enjoyed creative pursuits and had recently taken up learning how to play the ukulele as a fun pursuit. I knew Campbell had recently received her latest report card, and she was thrilled with her personal progress. Her parents were also happy about her academic performance but admitted they had called the meeting because they wanted their daughter to push herself even further. "We know she can do it," they exclaimed. In their attempts to motivate Campbell, they asked her how she could make those B+'s into A's. Hearing that made me wince—I knew what was coming next. The intended inspirational speech back-fired, and their daughter now seemed sullen, withdrawn, and seemingly unmotivated. Retelling the story, the parents sat in my office, dumb-founded as to why. After all, they clearly believed in her and thought they were being encouraging.

There's nothing wrong with encouraging excellence and believing in continuous progress and improvement. But Campbell's parents' focus on numbers achievement had the negative effect of making her want to give up. Campbell was happy with the progress she was making as she became more mindful of her efforts inside and outside the class-room. She was developing an intrinsic motivation pulled from her own evolving personal values. Her parents' reaction made her feel as though nothing were ever good enough and that any additional efforts would be met by underlying criticism. At that point, why bother?

Even in our modern child-centric world, parents and parental figures can still dominate a girl's developing outlook. For a school-age girl, shaping influences can filter in from all sorts of unpredictable di-rections: from the cultural cosmos to the social spheres of friends and peers to the microcosm of the individual school or classroom. Some-where near the core of these constellations are her parents or the adult role models who play a parental role and the home life she and they create together. And because parental figures are just as susceptible to having their views shaped by the achievement culture as their girls are (indeed, many parents have grown up with these pressures themselves), they also run the risk of unwittingly promoting patterns of success in their daughters that can exacerbate the filling-the-box phenomenon. Parents can do so by detrimentally focusing on their daughter's external accolades and achievements, whether that success is in school, on the playing field, with friends, or within the community.

It is natural for parents to want a better life for their children— whether *better* is defined quantitatively as access to educational or extracurricular opportunities or qualitatively as more time spent as a family or improved parent–child relationships. But we often need to remind ourselves that our children are not necessarily a reflection of us and that laying out set, defined expectations or creating double-edged valuations—"I know you will make the varsity water polo team" or "You can be a 4.0 GPA student"—can be stifling, limiting, and somewhat counterproductive. Often parents don't even realize that the unintentionally overbearing expectations they put on their children can be the impetus for underlying emotional damage because the children end up equating feeling loved internally to performing well externally.

Role Models Are Closer Than They Appear

Most parents agree that today's children are deeply influenced by the media, sports figures, friends, and peers, even by the reality-show winners and losers who seem to become part of the family. What many fail to realize, however, at least explicitly, is that parents and parental figures are often still the most influential people in their children's lives. This is an obvious fact but it needs to be emphasized precisely because the odds seem so stacked against parents. Indeed, girls can seem so determined to find fulfillment elsewhere that it can be difficult to assert the governing authority that you still do in fact possess. It is easy to incrementally abdicate parental responsibility as girls become immersed in popular culture or when modern work life makes it almost impossible to think about being the parental mainstay you thought you would or should be.

Even so, you can each sort out your own priorities and promote habits that make you happier. And that means being open to reflecting on the actual patterns of behavior you follow rather than merely on what you say and to examining your own motivations, hopes, dreams, and anxieties. Being hurried and never fully present at one task, either at work or at home, may seem to instill lessons about climbing mountains, breaking down barriers, and achieving great things. But it also sends messages about how you value different kinds of engagement.

A good example of parental influence is driving and texting. The majority of states have a ban on sending text messages while driving, and overwhelming research shows that distracted driving contributes to accidents. While many parents talk about the dangers of texting and talking on a cell phone while driving, many don't realize that their own behaviors with technology are contributing to the craze. In fact, 2009 research from the Pew Research Center shows that while 24 percent of teenagers admitted to texting while driving, a number of the teens in focus groups reported actually being scared by their parents' driving behavior.

"They would tell stories about their parents texting with the phone while trying to drive with their knees," researcher Amanda Lenhart noted. "They would talk about other ways in which parents were distracted behind the wheel, including using GPS or trying to use the walkie-talkie function on the phone, or making calls."[2]

It's easy for parents to suppose that their sullen preteen or adolescent daughter isn't watching their every move because in some cases they may get little more than a one-word answer to an open-ended question. In actuality, though, most girls are thoughtfully observant, and their parents' behaviors and actions speak louder than their words ever could.

More than a few students have told me how awkward it is to see their parents' intoxicated behavior—parents are, after all, usually embarrassing while completely sober, so adding alcohol to the mix can be downright humiliating. But negative role modeling doesn't have to be as severe as drug and alcohol abuse. It can be as simple as the way you value yourself, the way you treat others, and the way you treat your time.

GIRLS ARE MORE ATTENTIVE THAN WE THINK

We often forget that positive self-reflection begins at home. With all the outside forces competing for our girls' attention, it is small daily interactions that can sometimes be the most meaningful. It's not only about weight or appearance but also about how we react to setbacks, face new opportunities, and embrace unexpected challenges and possibilities.

Reflect for a moment on the messages you are sending about weight, appearance, and the need to be it all and have it all. What are your own values? How do you define success? Is success defined in monetary gains, personal accomplishments, or other attainments? Think about a recent setback—big or small—how did you react? Are you sending healthy messages or ones that create a bubbling over of self-criticism and self-contempt?

EXERCISE

This exercise can be done by yourself or with the girl in your life. Create two lists. On the first list, write down all the things you like about yourself and about your life. On the other list, write down all the things that you want to change or are critical about yourself. *Notice which list is longer.* Where are you being unreasonably harsh on yourself? Where can you be nicer to yourself? Even if you haven't said anything aloud, how do you think your overall perspective affected your daughter's outlook on herself? Is there anything you would want to change about your influence?

ENTITLEMENT IS A LEARNED TRAIT

In my conversations with teachers and school administrators, I hear similar stories of parents who try to excuse their kids from homework policies, bad grades, or disciplinary action. For instance, a few years ago, five girls were caught drinking alcohol at a local school dance; they had created a classy mixed-drink cocktail in some plastic water bottles and were passing them around. When the vice principal caught them, the girls faced routine disciplinary action that included two months' suspension from all extracurricular activities, including athletics. Two of the girls were varsity soccer players and were in the process of being recruited by colleges. It was midseason, the playoffs were coming up in less than a month, and being suspended could clearly hurt their long-term chances. The parents decided to wage an all-out war. First, the parents actively tried to pin the blame on the three nonathletes, hoping that those girls could take the punishment so their girls could play and not see their athletic opportunities jeopardized. When that didn't work (and likely made school lunchtime seating arrangements somewhat strained), the parents brought in lawyers and had meetings with many high-level administrators—to no avail. The school stood its ground, but not before the girls were treated to a front-row seat to their parents' show of self-importance.

Separating Your Dreams from Your Child's Reality

A wonderfully loving and by all appearances nurturing mother I worked with a few years back had never had the opportunity to play the piano when she was growing up, and began taking piano lessons as an adult. She then encouraged (well, *encouraged* would be too gentle a word; it was more like *forcefully requested*) her three children to take music lessons as well. And so they all took piano lessons in perpetuity, even though only one of the children actually enjoyed it. Over the years, other activities filled the children's schedules, and piano playing filtered down to the bottom. Getting the kids to practice became a constant battle, and the weekly lessons were painful for all involved, especially the teacher who had to listen to the results of minimal practicing from one week to the next. It was really a needless struggle; the kids were all well adjusted and engaged in a number of activities they liked. The inclusion of piano was contributing to their becoming overscheduled. But when the oldest daughter, then a high school sophomore, asked to drop piano permanently, her well-intentioned mom countered, "Well, okay, but what about taking up choir? It's so important to have a musical background."

Telling me the story, the young girl looked a bit deflated. She played two sports and was heavily involved in activities that often occupied her until late in the evening. Piano was taking up the little free time she had on the weekends, and it didn't bring her a sense of enjoyment or joy that might have marginally justified its place in her already packed schedule. She evaluated her position and decided to confront her mother's wishes. But her mother was temporarily blinded by a desire to make sure that her children didn't miss out on the opportunity to be musically inclined.

When children are younger, it can be natural to sign them up for activities based on what their friends (or your friends) are doing. It can be a relief to sit next to people you like during long innings of T-ball or the four-hour band recital. And children do need to be exposed to lots of options, to see what they enjoy and might have an affinity for. But, given such license, it can be easy to fall into the trap of replacing experimentation with wish fulfillment, and pushing your child to do what you loved or wished you had done. Your daughter may be a bit of a pleaser and go along just because it's what she thinks you want. It requires a good deal of *parental* self-awareness, therefore, to preserve the daughter's exploratory freedom. Just because she has been taking dance lessons since first grade and is good at dance doesn't necessarily mean that she needs to continue through high school, especially if she no longer enjoys it and has other activities that now take up all her free time. Dogged obedience to an old pursuit may actually stifle her from figuring out her evolving interests. Even more detrimentally, by insisting on keeping up appearances, parents inadvertently encourage girls to focus on credentials rather than engagement and enjoyment.

It is also ironic how much of this behavior does not actually come from parents themselves. Parents often tell me that they encourage their daughter's continued involvement in an activity, even consciously promoting it at a serious level long after their child has ceased to enjoy it, simply because that seems to be what college admissions officers are looking for. But this is an illusion. It's true that colleges (and workplaces) look for engaged, committed individuals, but they also look for individuals who are readily able to adapt and grow and try new things in our ever-changing world and who are not burned out by life at seventeen. They want young people who are comfortably authentic in knowing who they are and what they are truly interested in, not individuals who are afraid to change and adapt as new opportunities become available. I think the trend will continue to swing in the other direction: as colleges have adapted to the somewhat artificially inflated, commitment-heavy applicants of recent times, they increasingly recognize the value of self-management and fullness as a person. Indeed, they already do.

EXERCISE

As a way of stepping back from your own investments in your child's activities, try this exercise. Write down the activities you enjoyed when you were younger. Now write down the activities that you wish you had been involved in or wish you had been better at when you were younger. Reflect on the activities your daughter is involved in. Are there similarities? Differences?

Now, think about the activities that make up the bulk of your schedule and your daughter's weekly schedule. Do you think those activities reflect her own interests and bring you or her a sense of pleasure and purpose? For your daughter, how many of those activities are rooted in the fact that they will look good on the college application?

Hand-Holding and Helicoptering

It starts out with a little editing on a language arts paper for her elementary school class. Maybe your daughter's fingers don't type as fast as yours, so she dictates as you type. And as you do, you make a few changes and suggestions along the way. As the years go by, you enjoy spending the time helping with homework or providing support on projects, so you overlook the fact that you have now done the majority of that science diorama or English presentation. Maybe you aren't the one giving the extreme amounts of help; it might be a tutor or relative or even a teacher. Whatever the case, debilitating hand-holding, by which a student gets the message that correctness is more important than learning, has increased in recent years. This increase is due, in part, to an increased focus on grades, scores, and standardized tests and is massively enabled by the increased reach of technology. At the same time, the increased participation of parents in every aspect of their girls' lives leaves many girls without the opportunity to develop their own critical thinking and reasoning skills.

In recent years, the term *helicopter parents* has been used to describe parents who are so involved in their children's lives that they seem to always be hovering right overhead. College deans and faculty use the term to describe parents who try to take an active role in their adult children's academic, social, and housing options long after these young adults have registered to vote and had their first legal drink of alcohol.

Well-intentioned parents often turn to maniacal helicoptering out of a displaced combination of care and fear. They truly care about their children and are afraid of some drastic consequences of their child making the wrong decision or getting the wrong grades. In some cases, their behavior might be a reaction against the more hands-off parenting they experienced in their own lives. Often they worry about having their kids experience the healthy disappointment that comes with living an active life. Some helicopter parents mistakenly view parenting as yet another achievement and believe that their children are direct reflections of their own parental skills. Consequently, any deviation from preset standards of excellence could inherently be seen as a parenting failure.

Unfortunately, though, the level of micromanagement that goes into helicopter parenting is actually disempowering to children. When a child is micromanaged, she gets the message that her own parents think she is incompetent. Micromanaging parenting styles also fuel the constant need for external validation that often leads to box-filling behaviors. Girls who have long been micromanaged have a tough time figuring out how to navigate waters on their own because they have always been guided by others, and somewhere along the way they lost the oars that would enable them to paddle out on their own. These girls continually look to others for input and validation instead of thinking for themselves and creating their own world based on their own vision, in part because they never developed trust in their own abilities. In college, it can also result in students having a more difficult time making the transition from high school to living away from home. Students who have been micromanaged can be less likely to reach out and engage in their new environments because their adjustment skills have been severely limited—their parents have soothed over the rough edges for far too long! Consequently, they may remain in close contact to home: calling, texting, emailing home many times a day, asking for advice about minutiae decisions, and/or coming home on most weekends, all at the expense of adjusting to their new environment away from home.

TECHNOLOGY AND THE ART OF MICROMANAGEMENT

Many adults can recall that boss or supervisor who made their life miserable. Maybe this boss was cold, calculating, and full of harsh criticism. Maybe this boss micromanaged every little moment and made subordinates feel as though they needed to defend taking a bathroom break. Soon after graduating from college, I had a boss who regularly left voicemails and sent emails marked "Urgent" at all hours of the day and night, on weekends, and especially on holidays. His definition of *Urgent* was exceptionally broad, including what most would regard as mundane or routine. Needless to say, very few people lasted long in that office.

With technology, the temptation to be the bad boss is ever greater. Surveillance, micromanaging, and inflexible rule dictating are now simple to implement; it can take an uncommon degree of humanity *not* to require that everyone be subjected to strict by-the-book adherence. More and more schools use online systems to post assignments and track grades and performance in class. School administrators argue that the benefits are universal: Students can check forgotten assignments, parents can see at a glance how their child is doing, and teachers can potentially spend more time preparing and teaching classes rather than wading through student and parent inquiries.

But the reality is often quite different from this lofty vision. In my experience with many students, the only universal effect is that online systems tend to create a heightened sense of anxiety. Some teachers don't update class information routinely; others post homework assignments late in the evening that are due the next day; what I call "stealth homework posting." Some systems spit out email notifications for each update; this generates a lot of nervous excitement about potentially substantial but usually minor news. Some parents admit that they check the online system daily. Problems ensue when they take on the task of monitoring the student's performance in virtual real time. Put in the position to micromanage, it is the rare parent who has the wisdom and willpower to refrain from interfering, step back, and preserve the student's private realm of responsibility. Imagine you are a girl whose school day was punctuated by a fight with your best friend and the revelation that the boy you like asked someone else to the dance. You sit down to a casual family dinner, only to be greeted by the question,

"So, dear, why did you get a seven out of ten on that pop quiz on *The Great Gatsby* today?"

For parents, resisting the urge to go online regularly (or even worse, getting automatic email updates whenever something is posted online) may take a significant effort. But ask yourselves what your ultimate goal is behind the constant checking up. Your daughter's grades and performance are her own. For junior high and high school students, you should have access to the online systems to see if anything is amiss (especially if your daughter is someone who doesn't like to reach out for help) because dramatic grade fluctuations could be the sign of a range of other issues. But step back and work with her to come up with a collaborative strategy if you feel like you need to keep a watchful eye. Limit your online check to once or twice a week, at set and regular times, and in her presence.

BRIBERY, BLACKMAIL, AND OTHER ARTIFICIAL INCENTIVES

Over the years, parents have told me about their various techniques to encourage their children to get better grades or excel athletically or otherwise. "Pay for A's," as one mother called it, or paying your daughter when she scores a certain number of soccer goals or taking her out to dinner when she runs a certain number of miles may seem to be encouraging excellence. But invariably, even when they work, these bribery techniques and external incentives prevent girls from developing their own intrinsic motivation. The girls' reaction to incentives actually ends up insulating them from exploring and determining their self-generated purposes and also, once again, perpetuates the notion that love is conditionally tied to performance of externally set expectations. And at the extreme, I can't think of a faster way to promote cheating and shortsighted box-filling behavior than to give children a potential income stream in this way. Think about it: you've promised your daughter an iGadget or a particular brand of designer jeans if she gets certain grades, scores, or achievements. In doing so, you've created an opportunity for her to potentially rationalize away ethical behavior in favor of achieving your preset expectations so she can receive said reward.

Girls are quick to figure out what will get them the results they are after and how to work the system, and a system of bribery can make these calculations all the more cynical. Instead of doing the hard work of developing and determining their own standards, the focus quickly shifts to the designer jeans or iGadgets they've been promised, and the rewards system quickly teaches them to abide by the bottom line.

When students come into my office for the first time, I have them set goals for themselves and think about their own personal vision. In terms of academics, I encourage students to focus on habits that they want to change rather than specific grade goals. This is what I mean by focusing on *meanings*: Targeting grades alone rarely leads to lasting change. Far more significant and durable is the confidence that comes from the experience of reflecting and working to change from the inside out.

I am fully aware that not every class in school is an intellectual awakening. But I also know that significant life lessons can occur if we change the way we view overall school experiences. Very often, as those underlying behaviors improve, so do grades and other numbers indicators, sometimes to heights that were once thought to be unreachable. The crucial point is that they improve because genuine understanding and skill have progressed, not because the student has somehow mastered the tricks of winning rewards. Confidence and optimism about actual life patterns regularly lead to academic improvements and have far greater impact than the quick ping of excitement that shortsighted bribes bring.

Who Else Plays a Valuable Role in Your Daughter's Life?

Though parents can be enormously influential in their children's lives, we also need to think about all the other adults who play a significant role in children's lives. As there are more and more single parent and two-income households, many girls spend a great deal of time under the care of people other than their parents. What messages do these individuals send through their words and actions? These caretakers are often major figures in the children's lives; it certainly behooves parents to be cognizant about the kinds of values these relationships are instilling. The key point is this: Most people ask prospective caretakers general questions about availability and experience with children but don't always inquire about the character of those who, in some cases, spend more waking hours with the children than the parents.

Who are the people who form the network of influential individuals in your daughter's life? This could include grandparents, aunts, and uncles who play a big role in her life or it could be a nanny or childcare provider she sees on a daily basis. Perhaps a coach or teacher or mentor plays a peripheral or more central role. What defines true character to them and what are their own personal values? If you don't know, it may be a worthwhile and interesting conversation to have.

Being a parent in today's world is extraordinarily challenging; to say that most parents are dealing with more than they bargained for would be an understatement. Taking a step back to realize the impact that your behavior can have in your daughter's developing outlook allows you to realize the enormous opportunity you have to promote positive change in both your lives.

Parents: Part of the Solution!

Tina and Joe are solidly middle-class parents who try to take an active role in both of their girls' lives. Tina is wiry and petite, with a shock of red hair and greenish blue eyes. Joe's olive complexion and dark features pay homage to his Guatemalan heritage. Tina is the sixth of eight children, and Joe also comes from a big family. While growing up, both had very little day-to-day interaction with their parents. With their own two daughters, Tina and Joe try to be supportive and loving parents, and they admit that they haven't had role models to live by, so sometimes they feel as though they are winging it. Tina is a nurse and Joe is a firefighter, and they are proud of the life they have created for their family. Joe loves his job, and Tina enjoys hers but is sometimes prone to reflection about other possible paths: "Was it my dream job? I don't know. I didn't get the chance to think like that—I needed a career to support myself, and being a nurse is a solid one."

Like most parents, Tina and Joe care deeply about their daughters' overall happiness. From their own lives, they understand the importance of practicality, but they are also determined to provide some of the wider-ranging support that they missed from their own upbringings. Trying to balance these wishes, however, they have been struggling with their older daughter, Allison, who has had trouble in school socially and does much better with adults than with kids her age. Allison's passion is knitting, which she has been doing seriously since she was five years old. For her, it is a way to relax and quell the anxiety that caused her to engage in self-destructive behaviors in the past. With the help of a therapist, Allison has begun to talk more openly about her fears and desires. Recently, this led to the revelation that someday she would like to own and operate a fiber farm, where she could raise and shear animals humanely, to create and sell a variety of fibers and yarns for knitting. Allison had done some pretty extensive research on fiber farms and actually found a place where she could intern for a few weeks over the summer.

"I was in shock," Tina said, relating the story to me. "I wanted to be supportive and happy that she was enthusiastic about something, but in the back of my head I was thinking, how in the heck is she going to make any money doing that?"

Tina went on to admit that when she was her daughter's age, her vision of appropriate careers was strongly limited to a narrow range of standard options. Though she clearly wanted her daughter to be happy, and had a kind of wistfulness in her own case about things she might have done, she had no concept of the feasibility of Allison's dream. How could it possibly work? Doesn't happiness require a firm foundation in the basics first?

What I want to say in response is yes, by all means be practical. Teach your children the values of hard work and thoughtful self-reflection. Show them that action makes a world, while conceptualizing only sketches it out. But also dare yourself, on your daughter's behalf, to stretch your sense of what is proper, appropriate, or fulfilling. As parents and adult role models, we can introduce our children to new courses of action and thinking, and we can also show, by being willing to investigate such possibilities ourselves, that we really mean it.

Embrace All Possibilities

To help a girl see her choices, you could encourage her to try a new activity or to pursue her desired college major, even if you were once convinced that it provided no future job options. It might be hard to bite your tongue and watch your child chase a dream that may or may not pan out. But part of what you're teaching when you *don't* lay down the veto is that opening ourselves to change not only makes us vulnerable to failure but also makes us responsive to purpose and excellence.

Loving girls just as they are, with all their strange and wonderful home-made notions, is part of actively freeing them from being dependent on outside expectations.

EXERCISE

The point of this exercise is to open yourself to understanding how ever changing our world is and how there are constant innovations creating new opportunities and possibilities. Either with your daughter or by yourself, sit down with a blank piece of paper and set a timer for five to ten minutes. Think back when you were half your age (so if you are forty-six years old today, think back to when you were twenty-three). List the things that exist today that would have seemed crazy back then. List the things that now exist that make your life better. (Swiffer dusters and GPS navigation would be on my list.)

Focus on Long-Term Efforts Rather Than Short-Term Results

During October of my freshman year in college, I was pretty devastated after receiving the results of my first midterms. I had completely failed my calculus exam (if memory serves me correctly, my *curved* score was somewhere in the thirtieth percentile), and had received a D+ on my first chemistry exam. I called home upset, and in a matter of moments, my frustration gave way to all-out tears. What if the admissions office made a mistake? I asked my father gravely. What if I am not good enough to be here?

My dad would have none of it. He calmly reasoned that these were only the first exams, and that I simply needed to adapt to my new learning environment. Sensing my weariness, he advised me to relax and take care of myself for the rest of the day. Once I was calmer, I could then carefully determine why I got each question wrong and could step-by-step begin to develop an entirely new study routine for the next set of tests.

I spent a fair amount of time in office hours and extra one-on-one tutorials in the following weeks, and ended the semester much better than I started. In time, I gained confidence from the new approaches: Figuring out how I could best understand the material became a central element of learning it in the first place. Instead of panicking when things didn't turn out as planned, I learned to reevaluate, reflect, and redirect future efforts. Most important, I learned a crucial lesson from my father's calm wisdom: It isn't the initial results but the longer-term habits and outlooks that really matter.

We can't always control the results, but we can control how we respond and react to them. It is easy to forget in this achievement-focused world the crucial lesson that allowing for failure actually stimulates growth. Especially in a world that emphasizes winning above all else, we often forget to praise the longer-term preparations that typically yield the success. But effort is a variable that girls can control and is one that we need to acknowledge much more directly.[3] Promoting a solid work ethic toward pursuits of personal interest, despite initial obstacles and entirely aside from whatever immediate rewards there might be, is ultimately one of the most productive things we can do for girls.

> It is easy to forget in this achievement-focused world the crucial lesson that allowing for failure actually stimulates growth.

In my office, students will sometimes become dismayed when they don't see immediate academic results from adopting my suggested organizational practices. To me, it's even sadder when a parent whose child has been making significant, albeit incremental, progress calls to complain that the improvement isn't happening fast enough. Genuine change takes time. Almost invariably, when parents and students reflect over a longer period—six months to a year—those who have stuck with a plan are astounded by their overall progress.

Results often take time, and young people generally think in the here and now: *Why didn't this happen yesterday?* This attitude is partially developmental but has also been magnified by our fast-paced society. We can now get information and answers in a few seconds that before might have taken hours or days, and we can easily fall into the trap of demanding that all results be that immediate. As the adults in our girls' lives, we need to step back regularly and model the patience that many of them are still developing, focusing on the long-term efforts rather than the short-term results.

REDEFINE AND REEVALUATE SUCCESS

What does success look like to you? Does success mean academic achievements, athletic accolades, or other accomplishments? Is it tied to money or social status? Is your definition of being successful a result of developing personal values and a moral code of ethics? Is it any or all of the above, or something completely different altogether?

In today's world, children are constantly sent the message that being extraordinarily overachieving is crucial for being labeled a success. Unfortunately, this definition creates a narrow window for success with standards that only get more rigid and unobtainable.

Take a few moments to think about how you define success, and what messages you send on what being successful looks like. Is your definition narrow or broad? Does it include more qualitative characteristics, like values and ethics, or quantitative characteristics, like scores and numbers? When we give narrow, defined versions of success that are focused on merely extraordinary accomplishments and accolades, we often overlook the ordinary, simple values and pleasures that bring us happiness and contentment. When we are younger, we appreciate the ordinary experiences: going to the park, reaching the top of the jungle gym, having a picnic outside, or eating birthday cake. Those ordinary, everyday experiences that can bring such simple pleasures often get lost in our achievement arms race, and much of why girls tend to think they are never good enough is because what was once the window to success has become a mere sliver or crack.

Allow Girls to Become the Creators of Their Own World

Karen was a well-connected mid-level manager at a local technology company. Her daughter Adrianna, then a college sophomore, was looking for a summer job and knew that a lot of her friends had found jobs and internships through their parents' efforts. When Adrianna approached her mom about helping her find a job, Karen replied with loving directness, "Adrianna, you can find yourself a better summer job than I ever could." At first, Adrianna was irritated that she now had to do more legwork than she initially thought she would have to. After mulling it over, she went to her university's career center and learned how to brush up her résumé and create a compelling cover letter. She searched the alumni database and sent out several thoughtful, personalized emails to graduates who were working in careers that interested her, asking about potential summer internships. She polished her interview skills by taking a workshop and doing a few mock interviews through the career center. A few of the alumni responded to her well-researched and well-thought-out inquiries, and ultimately Adrianna landed a paid summer internship in a field she found interesting that was far from her mom's network of connections and expertise. That internship led to a permanent job offer after she graduated and, more than that, launched Adrianna into her postcollege life as someone with the confidence to look to her own capabilities first.

Now, in our current economic state, there are more and more

parents who are taking an active role in their children's employment search. A 2012 article in *SmartMoney* magazine described the recent trend of parents taking over their children's job search, writing cover letters, sending out résumés, and in some painfully unfortunate cases, going along with them on the job interviews.[4] It's easy to want what is best for your child, and clearly these parents had good intentions (though why a parent would think it is okay to show up at a job interview to make sure the child "got a fair opportunity at the job" is hard to fathom). But it doesn't have to be as extreme as writing your child's cover letters. If you want your daughter to be a builder of her own world and find and define her own sense of personal purpose and develop a healthy intrinsic motivation, it is crucial to step back and allow her to develop her own.

One of the most freeing things you can do as a parent is understand and accept that your child, like you, is an imperfect person with faults, struggles, and challenges. We all are. Unfortunately, we have become too comfortable with shielding our children from the disappointments that should be a natural part of everyday life. In doing so, we inadvertently inflate the failures. When we allow girls to experience typical hardships and disappointments, we ultimately support them to become more resilient and powerful individuals. But when girls haven't developed the resilience that comes from picking themselves up and moving on, they can exaggerate and personalize the frustrations. And while it can be extremely painful to watch your daughter experience adversity, go through hardship, or do something wrong—especially if it is something that you know you could fix—perhaps it is comforting to know that by letting her experience the challenges of growing up you are allowing her to build herself up.

Of course, there are times parents should and need to be involved; and indeed, it is incredibly tough to find a comfortable balance with girls, who are less likely to be open about the challenges they face. And I am not saying that your daughter shouldn't necessarily use your connections, but that she should be the one making the phone calls, sending the emails, and setting up the meetings, not you. Realizing that a healthy vulnerability to disappointments is not something that needs to be controlled or avoided out of fear is a valuable lesson.

EXERCISE

As a parent, reflect on times when you have done something for your daughter that she could have dealt with herself. Perhaps you emailed the principal about a social issue or let the teacher know that your daughter was sick. How could you have given her the tools and resources to deal with the challenge and have taken a less active role yourself?

In the coming chapters, you will find exercises to help girls start breaking down the boxes and move into becoming more active rather than passive in their own lives. Resist the urge to offer external validation other than support and encouragement. Always ask for your daughter's thoughts and opinions first, and resist judgment in favor of expanding your own worldview and opinions. Use your ideas to expand your own limits and allow her to do the same.

CHAPTER FOUR

Breaking Down the Boxes

A few weeks after I gave a talk at a local public school, Maggie's mom called our office asking for a consultation. Maggie was an incoming high school junior, and her mom wanted me to look over her transcript and give suggestions for general goals, plans, and classes for the next year. But when the three of us met, Maggie, as it turned out, had a lot of her own concerns. After talking with her friends, she said, she frequently worried that she wasn't taking the right classes to get into the right college. While her mom sat by silently, Maggie reeled off a list of in-depth questions, anxieties, and fears. It didn't take me long to figure out that, in addition to her worries about her future, Maggie was academically overwhelmed: She was taking mostly advanced placement (AP) classes, and her homework regularly kept her awake late into the night, sometimes all night. She admitted that she spent hours poring over college websites and brochures, talking with other friends (real and virtual) online about the pros and cons of different colleges, and trying to figure out what each was looking for. It was a surreal and almost hilarious image: a conclave of digital personalities debating into the wee hours over admissions policy minutiae of tiny liberal arts colleges in

Maine. But Maggie was deadly serious and deeply anxious—what she really wanted was for me to tell her exactly what she should do in order to get into the right college.

And that's where I stopped her. "Like the universal definition of *beauty*, Maggie, there is no one right answer now, and there never will be."

With that, our conversation turned. We began to talk about what she enjoyed, and then about what she could cut from her schedule to create more time for her own enjoyment and personal interests. Initially confused, she became increasingly animated when I suggested that pursuing more of her own interests and taking a less one-dimensionally work-intensive route might be a healthier, and in fact more productive, option for her. She admitted that when she was exhausted ("Ana, I spent my entire sophomore year sleep deprived!") she was irritable, sluggish, and unable to do anything well, which just left her feeling increasingly overwhelmed. As a first step, I encouraged her to identify three things she enjoyed, for their own sake, and for her that was baking, going on long walks with her dog, and taking a bath. We also talked about the organizational and time-management techniques (highlighted in Chapter 5) that would help her find an extra few hours in her week.

Maggie was receptive to the idea and promised to try this little experimental loosening. But what struck me most in this meeting was how much Maggie's mom wanted to hear me tell her daughter to take fewer AP and honors classes. This mom could readily see that her daughter was becoming a shell of the exuberant, vibrant young girl she once was.

Over the next year, Maggie followed through and took one fewer AP class and managed her time so she regularly got eight hours of sleep per night. Even though she was still taking challenging classes, she felt both more relaxed and fuller in her life; she could sometimes read for pleasure, or spend a few hours on Sunday baking with her mom, or take the dog for a long walk on a Wednesday evening. Her interest in computer science was piqued by her volunteer work at the food kitchen through her local church—she helped develop a system that reduced food kitchen clients' wait time for bags of groceries from an hour to less than ten minutes. She saw the way her efforts gave dignity to those in need, and started to take computer science classes at the local community college to learn more. She enjoyed these things and did them just because she could: The motivation wasn't the ambition to have done them or to be able to add them afterward to a list of accomplishments. Rather it came from the experience itself, flowing from appreciation and interest.

This story has a happy ending, in both ways. Maggie enjoyed living more in tune with experiences that she thought were fun. She started to explore her sense of purpose through her work at the food kitchen and her interest in computer science. And, as I have found is often the case, she also flourished academically. In her senior year she gained admission to the college of her choice—not in spite of, or exactly because of, but beautifully in consequence of a healthier perspective on the integration of her school and life. She decided to major in computer science because of her genuine interest in the field and her understanding that she could use her natural abilities to develop her sense of personal purpose.

Goals and Purposes

In my first book, *That Crumpled Paper Was Due Last Week*, I wrote about goal setting. Setting goals is one of my favorite parts of my work because it gives students the opportunity to dream big and start to envision themselves moving toward something they silently wished for but were afraid to say out loud. Girls can sometimes be a little different in this area. Some of the girls I see, though of course not all, can set goals without a problem; it is one of the themes of this book that the challenge for girls is often in the other direction: that they fasten onto programs to achieve externally defined success too readily, and in fact go on achieving, achieving, and achieving some more, with little regard for their genuine preferences.

Setting goals can therefore be a tricky task with girls because they can develop such a razor-sharp focus on the process that they tend to overlook the bigger picture. Their goals are sometimes the rewards they think they should want rather than the enjoyment and pleasure they really need and deserve.

That is why, with girls, I like to talk less about setting goals and more about discovering their sense of *purpose* and *fun*. I ask them to think about setting purposeful goals that reflect their own values and greater vision of who they are and what they ultimately enjoy. It is important, in this reframing process, to encourage girls to use their own resources to find solutions for their own lives, and to create and build a world that is authentic to them. When girls realize that success is whatever they want to make of it, the idea of achievement softens and becomes empowering instead of overwhelming. In a sense, this work is even more fundamental than with boys, especially as girls enter the culture of female objectification. Instead of focusing on doing (painting a mural or finishing a marathon), I encourage girls to find the enjoyment in being (being an artist or being a runner) because the latter opens the opportunity to reflect on a personal state or stance, whereas the former can conjure up a to-do list that can slip quite quickly back into the whole scheme of filling the box, bit by bit or task by task.

Reflecting and developing purposeful goals can help girls become motivated about adapting many of the habits throughout this book. Parents often wonder how students who come to our office can sometimes get so quickly excited about adapting the organizational habits and promoting new possibilities. In truth, it is often because they are, for the first time, reflecting on what kind of life they really want to lead, develop, and discover.

PROMOTING PURPOSE RATHER THAN VOCATION

When children are young, they are often asked, "What do you want to be when you grow up?" It's an innocuous question, and some children readily give a long list of answers that change with regularity. Asking that same question of a teenage girl can provoke a sense of fear or anxiety. Though some may have a defined vision of what they want to do, many are unsure. Especially in economically challenging and ever-changing times, potential opportunities may be fluidly evolving. And so, asking a teenage girl what she wants to do with her life should become less a question of fixed vocation, and more of an encouragement of her own values' reflection.

In his thoughtful book *The Path to Purpose*, Stanford University professor William Damon explains his belief that schools don't place an emphasis or importance on helping students discover a future path that they will find rewarding and meaningful.[1] Consequently, students are often left to their own devices to try to find a sense of meaning without the guidance and support that can be crucial, and that is precisely the role parents and mentors can play. Damon defines the purposeful as those who have asked the tough questions to find the ultimate answers as to *why* they are doing something. They work to define something that is meaningful to them, a greater calling that is much more substantial than immediate goals and daily routines. Without a sense of purpose, young people are more likely to drift instead of finding deeper meaning to their work that extends beyond the here and now.[2]

Adolescence is such a critical time to figure out and develop one's sense of personal identity, and what can easily get lost in this arms race of achievement is the cultivation of self-reflection and self-awareness inherent to developing a personal sense of purpose. Authentically exploring and finding a sense of personal purpose is highly undervalued in a world in which it can seem to be all about getting into the right school or having the right stuff or landing the right job. But a young girl's foundational belief that she can have a monumental impact in her greater world through her meaningful engagement can have a remarkable effect on her overall outlook. There is a powerful link between the pursuit of a positive purpose and life satisfaction: Thoughtful and positive character development can be the result of recognizing and realizing a sense of personal purpose within our greater world.

Discovering a sense of purpose is a daring, yet altogether essential challenge for girls if they want to move beyond box filling and become builders of their own world. It requires them to step back and objectively understand their abilities and talents, and recognize what is meaningful to them, which can be extraordinarily different from what is important to those around them. This can be scary because the exploration process can leave them open to their own vulnerabilities and fears of failure and criticism. It seems easier to follow a predetermined path toward a certain job or career track than to ask the ultimate "Why am I doing this and why is it important to me?" questions.

But we all long for the happiness and contentment that comes from a life filled with meaning and intent and hope to find a greater purpose for our place in this world. When girls develop their sense of purpose, it can be translated to many different career options or opportunities; it actually expands their worldview rather than restricts it. Many girls are currently reaching the point at which they could potentially be asking, exploring, and answering these questions of why sooner, without the crucial support and encouragement that they need. Without guidance, such girls can give up in favor of box-filling behavior because the questions are tough and the answers are not always readily apparent. In a world in which girls may look to their peers and media outlets for guidance, an often overlooked but crucial concept is understanding that what brings personal purpose to one girl's life might be different from what fulfills others.

If we engage in the supportive pursuit of helping girls ask and explore what gives them a sense of pleasure and purpose in life, we take the first important step in helping them become the builders of their own world. It is natural for parents to want their children to do well, and sometimes in pursuing that desire it's easy to overemphasize finding a job over developing a sense of purpose. One of the reasons this can seem so overwhelming is that our current culture—through micro-celebrities, reality television, magazines, and social media—sends the message that our sense of personal self-worth should be defined and evaluated by what type of people or how many people readily respond to us. But it's not how many Facebook friends, Twitter followers, or YouTube hits one gets that builds long-term self-fulfillment; in truth, it's an inward exploration rather than a result of external validation. Most young girls today have grown up in a world where their development and understanding of their sense of personal purpose has been thwarted within the greater world, and we need to change that.

DISCOVERING PURPOSE AND INCORPORATING PLEASURE INTO REAL LIFE

The upcoming exercises ask questions about the interests that girls (and young women) want to include more of in their lives. As they go through the exercises, girls may get excited about the idea of incorporating more fun and personal interests into their life, or they may be slightly cynical and dubious whether they are ever going to find the time to do any of the activities they would like to try. After all, school and related activities may take up so much time. Using the tips in Chapters 5 and 6, girls can find some concrete tools to start allocating their time more efficiently so they are more readily able to incorporate this exploration and discovery process into their lives.

When students come into my office for the first time, I want to get a sense of how they spend their time. None of us can do it all, all the time; trade-offs must be made. I use the Time-Management Sheet (page 98) and the Weekly Flow Chart (page 100) to help girls visually understand where and how they are spending all those hours. Together, two exercises help girls start to think about how to reallocate time and incorporate more of what they want into their life. Even if it is only one to two hours of the week that they can spend outdoors or thirty minutes a day that they can spend mindfully on a craft project that they find enjoyable, that small shift in mind-set can plant the seed to make a much larger difference.

Time Management Sheet

The Time Management Sheet is a tool that helps girls start to look at what they are prioritizing in their lives. They create an overview of the number of hours they are typically spending on school, homework, and other activities, and then have the opportunity to reflect on how they want to be spending their time.

NAME: Susie's Time Management Sheet

Academic Commitments	Class Description	Hours Required per Week (Outside Class)
COURSES		
Math	Algebra II	4
Science	Biology	4
English	English 2	4
Social Studies	World Studies	4
ELECTIVES (including world language)	Spanish 2	4
	Ceramics	1
TOTAL HOURS IN SCHOOL PER WEEK		35

Other Commitments	Activity Description	Hours Required per Week
Sport(s)	Junior Varsity Tennis	12
Music, theater, art		
Community, family	Church Youth group	4
Job, work	Babysitting	3
Volunteer work	Volunteering at the pet shelter	4
Hobbies	Hanging out with friends	4
	Watching TV	3
Other (regular weekly appointments)	Tutoring	2
Preferred amount of sleep	8 hours each night	56
TOTAL HOURS IN ONE WEEK		168
TOTAL TIME COMMITMENTS WITH THIS SCHEDULE		144
TOTAL FREE TIME (subtract total time commitments from total hours in one week)		24

NAME: _____

Academic Commitments	Class Description	Hours Required per Week (Outside Class)
COURSES		
Math		
Science		
English		
Social Studies		
ELECTIVES (including world language)		
TOTAL HOURS IN SCHOOL PER WEEK		

Other Commitments	Activity Description	Hours Required per Week
Sport(s)		
Music, theater, art		
Community, family		
Job, work		
Volunteer work		
Hobbies		
Other (regular weekly appointments)		
Preferred amount of sleep		
TOTAL HOURS IN ONE WEEK		
TOTAL TIME COMMITMENTS WITH THIS SCHEDULE		
TOTAL FREE TIME (subtract total time commitments from total hours in one week)		

Weekly Flow Chart

The Weekly Flow Chart offers a way for students to further visualize the ways they spend their time over the course of a typical week. Though each week is probably a little different from the one before, mapping out a more or less typical

NAME: Susie's Weekly Flow Chart

	Monday	Tuesday	Wednesday
6:00 AM			
7:00 AM			
8:00 AM	School	School	School
9:00 AM	School	School	School
10:00 AM	School	School	School
11:00 AM	School	School	School
12:00 PM	School	School	School
1:00 PM	School	School	School
2:00 PM	School	School	School
3:00 PM	Tennis	Tennis	Tennis
4:00 PM	Tennis	Tennis	Tennis
5:00 PM	Tutoring	Pet Shelter	Tutoring
6:00 PM	Homework	Pet Shelter	TV
7:00 PM	Homework	Homework	Youth Group
8:00 PM	Homework	Homework	Youth Group
9:00 PM	Homework	Homework	Homework
10:00 PM	Homework	Homework	Homework
11:00 PM			Homework

week will reveal where girls could find pockets of time to include activities that they would like to incorporate more of in their lives. Simply blocking out two hours on a Sunday night to do something they want to do can be the first step to realigning their time with something that is of personal interest to them.

Thursday	Friday	Saturday	Sunday
School	School		
School	School		
School	School		
School	School		
School	School	Pet Shelter	
School	School	Pet Shelter	
School	School		
Tennis	Tennis	Homework	
Tennis	Tennis	Homework	
Tennis Match	TV		
Tennis Match	Friends time	Babysit	
Homework	Friends time	Babysit	Youth Group
Homework	Friends time	Babysit	Youth Group
Homework	Friends time		TV
Homework			
Homework			

NAME:

	Monday	Tuesday	Wednesday
6:00 AM			
7:00 AM			
8:00 AM			
9:00 AM			
10:00 AM			
11:00 AM			
12:00 PM			
1:00 PM			
2:00 PM			
3:00 PM			
4:00 PM			
5:00 PM			
6:00 PM			
7:00 PM			
8:00 PM			
9:00 PM			
10:00 PM			
11:00 PM			

Thursday	Friday	Saturday	Sunday

HOW TO USE THE TIME MANAGEMENT SHEET
AND WEEKLY FLOW CHART

EXERCISE

Have your daughter fill out the Time Management Sheet and the Weekly Flow Chart (you can too, if you like!). She should fill out the Time Management Sheet first to get a sense of how many hours she needs to spend on schoolwork and other activities. This exercise should give her a breakdown of an average week. What optional activities does she think take up too much of her time? How could she change that? How can she shift things to get the ideal eight hours of sleep per night if she isn't already doing so? On the Weekly Flow Chart, have her block out several times per week to pursue personal interests and relax. This exercise can simply serve as a brainstorming guide and a way for your girl to see where her time is really going and where she would like it to go so she can start to have a more expansive view of her personal possibilities.

THE GAME OF THREES

After students get a sense of their schedule, I start the process of thinking about purpose and fun with a simple exercise that I call the "Game of Threes." Girls can do this on their own, or parents and teachers can easily use this at home or in the classroom to spark a conversation about dreams and personal interests that once seemed intimidating or too risky to pursue. Collaborative efforts are often the most effective; getting family members, friends, and classmates involved creates a supportive environment that creates a sense of accountability.

The first step in the Game of Threes is a brainstorming exercise. I have girls come up with three lists: things they enjoy doing, things they want to do more of but haven't been able to, and things they would like to try but haven't for whatever reason. I have included a sample worksheet on page 107. When I did this exercise with an eighth grader named Julia, her answers included "ice skating, fishing, baking" (what she enjoyed doing), "pleasure reading, journal writing, drawing" (wanted to do more of), and "photography, yoga, hip-hop dance class" (wanted to try but hadn't been able to yet). The second step is simply to choose three items from the set of lists and commit to making time for these three activities at least three times over the next three months.

Why three things incorporated at least three times over the next three months? Well, it's easy to remember (and a bit of a tongue twister) and it's also a nicely limited but still meaningful commitment. Three isn't an overwhelming number, but it still provides variety. If one idea doesn't work out for whatever reason, there are other options. *Three times* because it's important to try things more than once or twice to get a true sense of the experience. The first time someone takes an ice skating lesson or dance class, everything is so new that it may be hard to see beyond the details of technique. It's true that it may take more than three tries to get a full sense of a person's interest, but three is a good, reasonable start. If things go well, girls could ideally incorporate the activity weekly or so into their routine.

Why three months? As a deadline, three months gives enough sense of urgency without seeming overwhelming. It allows girls to spend time gathering information and exploring options if they want to try something brand-new. It's also a reasonable time frame for adjusting their schedules to include the new activity. In the life of a preteen or adolescent, six months or a year can be an incredibly long time; three months is long enough to explore options but short enough to allow for the normal evolution of interests.

What happens during those three months? Girls research and discover ways to incorporate their highlighted interests into their lives. Parents and others can play helpful roles with weekly check-ins as an encouragement for girls to see where they can block off two or three hours over the week to promote their chosen interests. Each girl is different, and the choice of support person can be important. An aunt, family friend, or older cousin may be welcome and appreciated as a mentor, more so than a mom or dad trying to give the same level of support.

What happens after three months? Girls should reflect to see what worked, what they learned, and what they would do differently. Some girls may decide to go through the process again. Some girls may really take to one of their new activities and wish to expand their commitment. Or maybe something else has popped up and displaces other items on the current list. As girls evolve, change, and grow, the Game of Threes can be repeated many times. Over an extended period, it can act as a kind of baseline for tracking, provoking, and inciting the adoption of new interests. It is a record of evolving engagement and can be inspiring and exciting for the girls as much as for anyone else.

What are some potential roadblocks and strategies to ensure success? Girls (and indeed most of us) sometime struggle with trying something totally new and can create roadblocks for themselves. Some girls are scared at the prospect of being uncomfortable or out of place. Others will say they don't have the time or money. But there are almost always alternatives that can work; use these excuses as opportunities for brainstorming further solutions. Ellie, a high school sophomore, wanted to try a yoga class but was nervous about running into someone she knew at the local studio. When I encouraged her to come up with alternatives that would help her comfortably reach her goal, she decided to take a class at a studio across town and go with a family friend. After a few months, she became much more comfortable and confident and started going to classes in her neighborhood as well as the studio across town that she had grown to love.

||||||||||||||||||||||||||||||||||||||||||||||||||||||||||||||||||||||||||||||||||||||||||||||||||||||||||||||||||||||||||||||||||||||||||

The Game of Threes

Create three lists: things you enjoy doing, things you want to do more, and things you'd like to try but haven't been able to yet. Next, circle three items from the lists and set time aside for these three activities at least three times over the next three months.

Things I Enjoy Doing	Things I Want to Do More	Things I Would Like to Try
1.	1.	1.
2.	2.	2.
3.	3.	3.

Active Living and Engaged Learning

One of the challenges in today's world is that we have such a buildup of what I like to call trophy confidence. Here's the problem: Someone telling a girl that she's awesome and giving her a proverbial trophy may make her feel better for a moment, but that moment is fleeting. After that initial high wears off, she may find herself searching for the next symbolic trophy—getting good grades, or doing what it takes to become socially accepted, or figuring out how to get into the right college or snag a job at the perfect company. As a result, a box-filling focus on external rewards and other people's standards of excellence can start to set in.

But true confidence doesn't come from winning the endorsement of others (though it is wonderful and important to feel appreciated and loved!). True confidence comes from *active* living and *engaged* learning.

Think about a time when you really mastered something that you once found daunting and maybe even impossible. It could be as simple as when you learned how to ride a bike, first wrote code for a web page, or completed a graphic design project. Maybe it's when you mastered making a soufflé or gave your first dinner party with ease. What made the difference was that you persevered. You had to contend with your inexperience before you could pass through it into capacity, mastery, and success.

Active learning is a three-dimensional process that involves being able to apply knowledge across contexts. Realizing how we learn best is tricky—what works well for one person might not work well for another. Classroom instruction doesn't always give students the time and space to figure out how they learn best because learning is an individualized process that can easily get lost in a room full of peers. Some individuals retain information best when studying in crowded areas, whereas others need to be in silent solitude. Some students learn best by simultaneously listening to and looking at information, and others benefit most from drawing pictures and being kinesthetically engaged in the learning process.

One of the most important tools we can give girls is the opportunity to master how they learn best. In doing so, they can gain confidence from understanding and developing their own personal learning style and becoming fearless learners both inside and outside of the classroom. Most students have to experiment to understand their particular learning style. Some girls can use what is being taught in the classroom as a guide for figuring out what they want to learn and how they can go about understanding the material. For others, lessons in active learning can take place outside of school. Regardless, girls who understand their learning process become empowered because they take charge of mastering material in the way that they see fit. Active learning is not, for instance, simply memorizing the names of states and capitals to satisfy the requirements of a geography exam. It is learning, understanding, and accepting how she learns best and being able to see the connections between a biology lesson on adenosine triphosphate (ATP) energy and realizing what she eats at lunch does really affect her energy level. Unfortunately, this type of learning can be easily lost in the shuffle of everyday life.

EXERCISE

Your daughter can try this exercise on her own or in parallel with you or others. It can build on the Game of Threes or stand alone as a separate exercise. The key questions are, What do you want to learn? And how can you learn it best? Have your daughter pick a few hobbies or activities that she has always wanted to learn. Examples from students who have done this exercise include learning how to make and edit a video, design a web page, use a DSL camera to create beautiful photographs, and sew or knit. Out of those listed, she should pick one item that is feasible within the constraints of her ordinary life (for example, learning how to fly a plane might be a bit tough for some to arrange, but learning to horseback ride is easy if there are stables nearby; brainstorming a full range of scalable options is important). There are no wrong answers, and part of the fun is coming up with unexpected possibilities. Unusual ideas are great, including many tactile hobbies. For example, knitting works well because it's relatively simple and approachable but also has many branches of skill, including math, counting, and figuring patterns.

Once the activity is selected, have your daughter come up with ways to learn it. Perhaps she can take a class, watch a video, or read a book. Have her experiment with methods and keep track of what works best. Was it easy enough just to pick up a book and follow the directions? Or did she need one-on-one guidance? Did she enjoy tactile instruction? Did she prefer taking a class where there was a community? Try several different ways of learning the hobby or different branches of it. With knitting, for example, she could follow a basic YouTube video to figure out how to cast on stitches and then get hands-on instruction at a local community class to learn the basic techniques. We all learn and work differently, and we all have our own way of absorbing and processing information. Some girls need more hands-on, kinesthetic interaction, while others process things best when they hear them. Still others prefer to see visuals or can do just fine reading a manual. The point is that everything is adjustable; everything is a reflection of the girl involved.

SOME POINTS TO KEEP IN MIND:

Explore alternatives. Encourage the girl to research multiple ways to learn the material as well as the different costs associated. For instance, if she wants to learn photography, remind her not to become fixated on the first method that comes to mind. Private photography lessons might be too expensive but a local studio might have a student rate or a local community center might offer beginning classes. Encourage her to try several different *styles*—online classes, model building, interviewing experts. Everything is up for consideration.

Keep the feeling of fun experimentation. Learning how you learn is exciting! When you figure out something about how you function best, it's as though you unlock a secret, and the power of that Aha! moment should not be underestimated. Have your daughter keep records of what worked, what didn't, what was funny, and what made the active learning exercise memorable. I have seen girls create mini-videos, PowerPoint presentations, and scrapbooks filled with photos that left me crying with laughter. Maybe you want to try to learn something new at the same time and record your journey as well. A little humor goes a long way toward making an experience memorable.

Be sure to have your student schedule time to devote to this process. Absorbing and understanding new material will not happen overnight. Consider overlapping with the Game of Threes; one of the items chosen in that exercise can be extended into this one. This exercise can definitely be an opportunity for parents and daughters to focus on something they have wanted to learn, either to do together or separately. And it needn't be scheduled during the school term; this could be an ideal way to give structure to a long summer break or vacation. Plan ahead. Background research might need to be done in advance, so consider planning on about a month of prep work to allow your girl to get the pieces into place.

FEARLESS LEARNING

A fearless learner is open to trying new things, taking healthy risks, and expressing her curiosity. She isn't afraid of failure and is excited to try something new that she might grow to love doing. She realizes that she doesn't need to be perfect or get it right the first time. Fearless learners welcome new opportunities, don't shy away from potential challenges, and are excited to learn for the sake of expanding their knowledge base. Their lives are full, interesting, and adventurous. Fearless learners are all about expansion and absorption. Many of us were like this when very young, which is why electrical socket protectors and baby gates were invented. But somewhere along the way—perhaps when we started juggling hours of homework with activities that felt more like a burden than a benefit—many of us lose that reckless love for the new. It is a trait that girls especially are not often encouraged to cultivate.

With the exercises in this chapter, there is no real limit of time, and they are meant as a way to encourage girls to expand their options, opportunities, and possibilities. Recognizing and understanding personal potential is a lifelong skill that benefits anyone who continues to develop it. Of course, some girls will quit their activities after experimenting with them a short while. That is fine and part of the process. The point is not necessarily to identify a lifelong pursuit in the first go, but rather to encourage an exploration and pursuit of personal interests. Your daughter can stop if she doesn't enjoy the activity; try something new, armed with the knowledge gained from the first attempt. An important caveat is to encourage girls to give a new activity enough time and effort to allow for the building of basic skills, because often activities become more enjoyable once basic skills are mastered. To maximize the chances of success, be sure she chooses something she actually wants (rather than *thinks* she wants or *should* want) to learn and help her break the activity down into simple steps that can be managed.

There really is no telling where the process might end because the kind of focus and energy expressed in the exercise are basic to any kind of passionate pursuit. One girl I worked with wanted to learn how to edit videos. She learned the basics by taking a local class and then a year later went to a summer camp devoted to the process. She is now majoring in film and production in college and just landed her dream summer internship working with a filmmaker. Like all real progress, it starts with little steps and, with diligence and energy, branches out from that base. Who knows where a girl's life can lead when she focuses on developing her own interests and sense of purpose?

The Entrepreneur's Model of Success

I started my first business—taking care of neighborhood pets—at the age of twelve. Even though I had only two regular clients, the confidence that came from running my own show was motivating and inspiring. When I started what would become Green Ivy Educational Consulting in 2001, I used some of the same strategies to slowly build that business. But it wasn't just the revenue stream and cost of goods and payroll issues that were important, though those were key. I took the opportunity to figure out the values that were important in my life—namely helping others, making a difference, being able to travel, having a somewhat flexible schedule, being my own boss—and worked to integrate them into my job. Starting from that foundation, I knew that whatever I built would be true to me.

I think such an opportunity can be usefully introduced, even to young girls, as a consciously adopted mind-set. The example I sometimes use to explain this idea to girls is Legos. In general, young boys play with Lego building blocks more than girls do, no doubt in part because of what they are expected to do by parents, marketers, and so on. The great thing about playing with Legos is that it offers the opportunity for building and rebuilding. (It is interesting that the Lego Group now offers products specifically marketed to girls, but those products do not have quite the same building and rebuilding qualities.) Children can try something out, and if it doesn't work, they make changes or start over from scratch. They make something that has never been made before. But the key is that they are building something with their own hands, to match a vision they have in their own heads. It's kind of a training ground for how to build your own world.

This is precisely the creative control girls should be able to assert over their own lives. The Entrepreneur's Model of Success aims to help them do just this. It tells girls: *You* can start from nothing and be the builder of your world, you can risk failure, and you can pick up the pieces again if it all falls apart and make something new and better.

Many young people have no idea what they want to do or what type of job they want to have when they grow up. And there is no problem with that. Indeed, many jobs that are sought after today did not exist even ten or twenty years ago. There are always girls who want to be a doctor or lawyer or engineer or other professional. But what does that really mean? What will they want their day to look like? Who will they hope to interact with regularly? What type of flexibility or structure do they desire? What motivates them to work? Many adult women wish they had thought more about these concrete issues before they launched themselves along certain career paths. Some figure these things out by trial and error after realizing how badly their first job failed to satisfy; it was only in the face of failure that the image of their desires came into focus. And none of that is inherently wrong, but giving girls the opportunity to start being conscious in their pursuits to envision a life full of what is important to them allows them to feel more confident and hopeful in their pursuits. Instead of being reactive, these girls can proactively work to create the life that is meaningful to them.

A college classmate of mine wanted to be a lawyer for as long as I had known her. She was a great student, graduated at the top of her class from a top law school, went to work as a corporate lawyer, and quickly became miserable. Though she performed well, she found herself going home at night frazzled, overwhelmed, and wondering why she was spending enormous amounts of her life on issues that for her were mundane and underwhelming. She was ill-suited for the job, and the job was ill-suited for her. The only upside was her paycheck, which wasn't as big as it seemed after student loan payments were deducted and after most of the rest of the paycheck went to relieving her stress. She left the law profession after only a few years and ended up teaching and working in a job at which she could use her talents and abilities and found pleasure and purpose in her work and life. Maybe going to law school was an important part of her journey, but a less circuitous and less expensive route would have been to ask the questions of personal purpose and pleasure earlier. For her, going to law school and working as a lawyer was really picked off the shelf as an achievement; it didn't grow organically as a result of thoughtful reflection.

A major contributing factor in some girls' passivity is a lack of confidence, whether intrinsic or learned, in their decision-making powers. More often than not, it can seem unwittingly easier to pick a predetermined path than carve one's own pursuit of personal purpose and excellence. When this is the case, it can be very useful to encourage a girl to take ownership of her own behavior and life path. You might well be a bit skeptical how someone who spends hours watching reality television and favors pants emblazoned with *Juicy* on her backside could become a builder of her own world. Sometimes the average fifteen-year-old girl can be hard to take seriously. But that would be a big mistake. Anyone who has worked with a determined teenage girl learns very quickly that there is very little that can stand in her way. The experience of being the boss of her own fate can jump-start the all-important goal of getting her proactively to think about herself and about building her own world.

EXERCISE

Have your daughter design her own dream business. The business can be an actual business plan for a business that sells goods and provides a service, but this exercise is more than just a way for your girl to figure out how to create revenue. It is designed to help her recognize her dream life, but to do so in a constructive, practical, and clear-eyed way. It asks her to start thinking about the details of who and what she would want to include if she were the boss, as indeed she is (or can be) in her own life.

With whom would she like to work? How would her work help others? Would she want to travel a lot? Live internationally? Work close to home? With whom would she like to collaborate? What kinds of personalities would she prefer to work with? What kinds of work might bring more of those people into her world? What effect does your daughter want her work to have on others? What values would she promote in her business life? Would it be important for her to interact with lots of people, or does she prefer solitude for creative or specialized work with bursts of interaction? Would she prefer constant change or a known routine? This exercise is designed to channel that determined girl energy toward personal and greater good. Naturally the answers to such questions will vary over time. But simply articulating her ideas in this framework can give much greater visibility to a girl who may never have thought of herself as owning and running her own show.

Not everyone wants to be an entrepreneur or to run a business, and that's fine. But we all *lead* our own lives, whether or not we acknowledge that fact. For many girls, it never occurs to them to stop, reflect, and take charge in a substantive way.

COMMUNITY SERVICE, SELFLESS SERVICE, AND FINDING PURPOSE

It has been only in the last few decades that many high schools have made community service hours a graduation requirement for students. Despite the best of intentions, this idea has, in many cases, backfired. Now, giving service is no longer viewed as something to be done simply because it's the right thing to do or because it brings a sense of personal fulfillment. Instead, community service has unfortunately become one more achievement to be competitively recorded and reported. It is now a commodity: In many cases, it is no longer the quality of students' experience but rather the quantity of their hours that counts. I wince when students ask how many hours of community service look good on a college application (and it happens more than I care to admit). Although there certainly are many students who tirelessly give their time and energy to causes they truly care about, the notion of selfless service has become rare when everything goes on the college application, résumé, or is in some way publicly acknowledged (or, in the social media sense "pics or it didn't happen").

Selfless service isn't necessarily the same as community service, especially when the service is done only out of obligation (that is, fulfilling a high school graduation requirement) or ulterior motives (thinking it will look good on college applications). Selfless service is openly giving without the expectation of anything in return, and its importance in personal wellness and development can be easily undermined in our achievement culture. There is a certain personal goodness and transformative quality we feel when we are of service to something greater than ourselves. Selfless service could be as simple as spending the

> Now, giving service is no longer viewed as something to be done simply because it's the right thing to do or because it brings a sense of personal fulfillment.

afternoon helping an elderly neighbor run errands, or pitching in at the local town parade when they are short-staffed. It could be a long-term project or a single day of service—regardless, it is the underlying interest and intention that makes all the difference. When girls are able to willingly participate in selfless service, their perspective expands. Doing something of benefit to more than themselves takes them away from their own troubles and helps them develop grace and gratitude.

Ultimately, selfless service is a way girls can begin to align their actions with their developing sense of purpose. It helps promote their own spiritual wellness and gives them the opportunity to start exploring what they are good at, and what they enjoy, and what brings meaning to their lives without the external pressure to achieve, accomplish, or produce.

EXERCISE

Have your daughter think about the community service she has done so far (if she has done any). Did she do it because she had to or she wanted to (or both)? What would she have done differently? Would she consider it selfless service? Why or why not? What feeling did she come away with (relief, annoyance, gratitude, joy)? What does selfless service look like to your girl? What is something she would do in service of others regardless of getting credit or recognition? What service would feel meaningful to her?

Taking the B

When Suzie came into my office, she was shaking with a nervous energy that resembled a twitch. Her short curly brown hair was somewhat disheveled, and makeup covered her splotchy skin. She couldn't keep from contorting her face into exaggerated expressions as she explained her schedule and her worries. It was clear that she was overwhelmed and stressed out. She was having a hard time keeping up with the home-work load for her classes and had just failed her English test and was struggling in Spanish class. Her parents were going through a divorce, and her older sister and brother had just left for college. She was trying to become a starter on her school soccer team, but an injured hamstring limited her chances. On top of that, there were social anxieties: Her friend group was going through some drama, and even though she was trying to remain aloof, it was draining her last energy reserves to empty with the red light flashing. After watching her organize her binders and listening to her narrative, I asked simply, "Are you doing the best you can with what you've got?"

Suzie stopped for a moment, and looked at me somewhat blankly. And then, after a thoughtful moment, she quietly responded with a simple yes. "Well," I replied, "that's good enough for now."

I told her to give herself the opportunity to take care of what she could and let go of the rest. Easier said than done, perhaps, but entirely feasible even in the most trying circumstances. Suzie and I used the following Taking the B exercise as well as some of the organizational strategies in the next chapter to help her prioritize her life so she could spend time on what she needed to do and Take the B on other things.

> I told her to give herself the opportunity to take care of what she could and let go of the rest.

Taking the B is not necessarily about grades or school, though for some girls it certainly should be. I mean it in two fun-damental ways. First, pragmatically, as a permission a girl can give herself *not* to have to achieve perfectly in every area. She can Take the B by allowing herself not to need an A, the better to get on with other things. It might be in a class that isn't cen-tral but is causing a lot of anxiety. Or it could be, as in Suzie's case, a complex life situation, where releasing pressure in one area will allow others to be attended to. But I also mean it philosophically, as an internal call to redirect her focus away from being boxed toward *being*—toward living actively on her own terms, in line with her own priorities.

This is an approach I use frequently with girls and young women to break down the mind-set of You Can Have It All, All the Time (discussed in Chapter 1). Taking the B involves tuning personal energy toward current purposes: What *she* needs and what *she* wants in school and life. There are many times when we cannot do it all, even when we know how it

> There are many times when we cannot do it all, even when we know how it all could be done.

all could be done. Too many girls feel like failures when they can't perform impeccably and end up anxious and overwhelmed as a result. It is, therefore, important to hear the emphasis I am putting on the word *taking*. This is a positive, power-inducing view. It is a means of restoring activity to the choices we make not to act in automatic, rote, or merely expected ways.

I've asked the question "Are you doing your best with what you've got?" countless times with students when they come in to the office stressed out and overwhelmed, either on the verge of tears or with tears freely flowing. It's a freeing question, actually; nobody's asking you to be perfect, and no one should be. It is also not asking for a girl's best effort because that varies with the ever-changing circumstances of life. Instead, Taking the B gives girls the opportunity to assess their efforts based on their current situation. If her grandparent is dying or her boyfriend just broke up with her or her family is in the middle of moving homes, she may not be able to handle the same workload as when school was going swimmingly and life was rosy. And that is perfectly okay. The only failure here would be to pretend that nothing changed when everything has turned upside down.

This shift in outlook might sound minor, but for girls who feel as though they've spent most of their lives climbing one ladder after another, reflecting one image of success after another, to make even a simple change in how they allow themselves not to compete can be truly liberating, and even profound. Most important, it can yield powerful results, allowing them to concentrate their efforts on what truly interests and motivates them, while Taking the B in other areas.

For some parents and educators, Taking the B will sound like a novel idea that would never work, in part because of the fear and anxiety surrounding the college admissions process. It's all well and good until Tania can't get into college, right? To fearful parents (and girls), Taking the B seems like closing off opportunities by paring down a schedule and reevaluating priorities, when in fact it is doing just the opposite. Taking the B is just one of many ways that girls can become ruthless prioritizers of their own lives and figure out the path that is in alignment with their vision and values. And girls who are able to actively start making those choices earlier are more attractive to everyone, including college admissions officers.

Some girls may be immediately open to figuring out where and when to allocate their energy resources; others will be somewhat terrified to think of easing off the throttle even for a second. Either way, parents really need to be involved in and support this decision-making process, especially for girls who are struggling with the idea of continual perfection. It can be part of an active conversation about general health, to ensure they are getting enough sleep, have a chance to relax, and are in emotional balance. After Suzie and I went through some strategies, I talked with both her parents about the notion of Taking the B and encouraged them to continue the conversation. At first, her businessman father was a little concerned ("Isn't she hurting her chances of college admission?"). But the idea resonated with him when I put it in business terms. Whenever resources are scarce, they need to be allocated efficiently instead of being overstretched and therefore underperforming. Taking the B allows girls to reevaluate and redistribute their own personal resources so they are optimal for the given circumstances.

EXERCISE

Using the Time Management Sheet from the beginning of the chapter, have your daughter look at where she might like to Take the B to redistribute her focus in school and life. A great way to start the conversation is to use the Weekly Flow Chart to see where she is currently spending her time and resources. Entire families can do this to see if their activities are in line with their personal interest and sense of purpose as discussed earlier in the chapter. Family units, too, can often benefit from reducing pressure in some areas to concentrate on what's really important.

Redefining Failure

In the past few years, an increasing number of teenage girls have told me they would love to try something but have resisted because they would only want to do it if they were good at it. One freshman girl refrained from trying out for the high school field hockey team because she was unsure of her abilities and then found out that many of the other girls who ended up making the freshman team were first-time players. These girls do well in school and from the outside they seem as if they have a healthy dose of confidence. And yet they avoid trying anything new and different for fear of failure, looking awkward, or feeling stupid. These girls have lost the adventurous risk-taking spirit of youth at an age when exploration is supposed to be a key part of their development process. When a girl hesitates to try something new out of a fear of failure, I often counter with the question, What's the worst that could happen?

In many cases, the worst-case scenario from taking a risk really isn't that bad. We need to redefine *failure*. It shouldn't be viewed as a failure if someone tries some-

> True failure comes from not trying.

thing and it doesn't work out, or if she shows up and finds that things don't go as expected. Instead, true failure comes from not trying, not having skin in the game, and not learning how to be adaptable and resilient.

EXERCISE

Ask your daughter to think of a few things she would like to try but has been afraid to. What were the reasons? How can those barriers be overcome or restrategized? For some girls, this exercise will build off the exercises earlier in the chapter.

Also, ask her to reflect on a time when things didn't go as planned or didn't work out. What did she do? Did that help or hurt? What would she do differently next time? How does that relate to her answers from the earlier exercises in the chapter? As a parent, you can do this exercise at the same time to make it a collaborative effort.

If we want girls to feel confident and empowered to explore and build their own world, we have to give them options for moving beyond the external standards and voices that can quickly drown out their personal efforts. In many ways, they have to embrace alternatives and ways of perceiving their own options and reality that allow them to focus on building their own individual world. It may be challenging, and there certainly is no one-size-fits-all approach, but I hope that in the upcoming chapters you will find strategies and suggestions that will work for your daughter and your family.

||||||||||||||||||||||

CHAPTER FIVE

Putting Purpose into Organizational Practice

When Maya first walked into my office, she seemed like she had it all together. She was articulate and personable, with neat binders and an organized planner. Her grades were good, and she spent most of her free time dancing, something she genuinely enjoyed. As we began talking, however, it became clear that she was driven and exhausted. Maya's mom was concerned that Maya was often up past midnight trying to complete her homework. Maya felt hopeless, thinking this was the way it had to be if she wanted to achieve. She assumed that her fate was sealed and that she was destined to remain sleep deprived, overcommitted, and unhappy.

"So, is your computer on when you do your homework?" I asked.

"Of course," she replied. Her teachers frequently posted assignments using the online school calendar, and most of her assignments required the use of the computer.

"And do your friends chat with you or send you instant messages? Do they know you're online?"

Again, Maya answered in the affirmative; after all, how else was she going to stay connected? If she was forced to spend countless hours doing homework late into the evening, sending texts and instant messages allowed her to keep up with the social scene at school even when she was buried in work.

"Maya, let's experiment for a week. For two hours a night, I want you to exit all chats and put your phone on silent in the other room. After those two hours, take a full half-hour break and then do another hour of work. After those two or three hours of work, see how much more you've gotten done and then feel free to chat and text all you want." I went on to share a few of the organizational strategies highlighted later in this chapter and told her about other students who had regularly gotten their work done an hour or two earlier than before. Her eyes widened as she promised to give it a real try. After all, there's nothing more enticing to a sleep-deprived teenager than the chance to have more time to sleep, socialize, and relax.

A week later, she admitted that my strategy had given her precious extra hours of sleep, without sacrificing her crucial social engagement opportunities. "Now, people know I am available after eight p.m.," she explained, which made it easier for her to disconnect before then and get her work done more efficiently.

Girls Need Organization Too

It never ceases to amaze me how deeply a few simple organizational changes can transform a student's outlook. When they feel out of control of the most basic elements of school life—Where is the assignment? What did I do with that essay? When is it due? How do I study for that test?—a student's functioning can devolve into a state of crisis management. Enormous amounts of mental energy are spent being confused, trying to hold everything together, and fighting off panic.

Conversely, a student who has a basic, effective system for keeping things in order, managing her time, and practicing good study habits is freer to think, work, and explore. Her brain is uncluttered by the constant feeling of unmet commitments, overwhelming schedules, and half-forgotten details. She can exude a sense of calmness and feels more in control of her possibilities, opportunities, and potential.

The focus of this book is not on organization per se but on how getting organized and being more efficient at directing resources of time and effort are crucial skills for *anyone's* success in school. Thus this and the next chapter set down some of the same practical advice I included in the chapters on organizational skills in *That Crumpled Paper Was Due Last Week*, my previous book geared for boys. Here I present the same kinds of easy-to-implement strategies, but my advice is condensed as befits my different emphasis. I hope the pair of chapters will serve as a toolbox—a one-stop tutorial or primer for those who want to think organizationally or for anyone who needs a friendly nudge back into orderliness.

Binders, Planners, and Other Essentials

Ashlee was a seventh grader who struggled socially at a local public junior high school. Ashlee's school counselor had referred her to our office because she sounded pretty dejected about school and life. Ashlee's mom was genuinely concerned for her daughter's overall wellness and said that Ashlee regularly missed homework assignments despite seeming conscientious. She had made very few friends in her first year of junior high. She wasn't doing terribly in school—she had mostly B's—but Ashlee's real story was her lack of confidence. When she came in for her first appointment, her head hung low and she could barely look me in the eye. Her one-word responses were so soft-spoken that I had to lean in to hear, and I eventually joked that my advanced age was affecting my hearing ability so she would have to increase her volume.

A few minutes into our first appointment, I asked if we could take a look inside her backpack. It became immediately apparent why school seemed like such an overwhelming burden. Her backpack was filled to the brim with crumpled papers—they almost exploded out of the bag when she unzipped it. Over the next two hours, we rummaged through the debris and found several near-empty binders that had not been used since the first week of school, a planner that remained untouched, and an assortment of textbooks. We must have sorted through close to four hundred pieces of paper, recycling some and organizing the rest into the binders. We sat on the floor and I offered background assistance while she sorted (and found a few bubble-gum wrappers and old comics in the process). In the end, she had a neat stack of binders, and every paper had a home. She smiled uneasily, as if she couldn't believe what just happened. But it was just the beginning of her transformation.

Over the next few months, one of my associates worked with Ashlee twice a week on developing organizational and time-management habits as well as on learning how to read and study new material—many of the same tools I introduce here. One day after school let out for the summer, Ashlee's mom stopped by our office to sign up for the next year and said, "Ana, I am not sure if you know, but Ashlee's grades improved in every single class. She got the best grades she ever has, but much more than that, she finally believes in herself, and her confidence has soared."

Indeed, when I saw Ashlee at the beginning of the eighth grade, she strode into our office assertive and prepared. Outside of school, she started to make friends at the local horse-riding stable where she took lessons and had a small part in the local community theater production. Even though she still didn't have a wide social circle at school, she had a group of friends to sit with at lunch, was looking forward to high school, and had found her main community of close friends outside of school. For Ashlee, as for many girls, the academic and the social were intertwined, and feeling confident in school helped her widen her social circle. In Ashlee's case, finding friends outside of school helped make her time inside the classroom more manageable.

BINDERS: A BULLETPROOF SYSTEM

Binders create a good, reliable system that captures all the loose papers, gives them a home for easy retrieval, and coordinates work material with a timetable for completion. In our office, we use a fairly simple and straightforward system for organizing binders. If possible, students should have *one* binder for each subject. In addition to being easy to remember, this helps to avoid *comingling*—the term I use when Spanish homework ends up in the front pocket of the history folder, and a frantic, rage-inducing thirty-minute search ensues. The goal of the binder system is for students to have all the material they need for each subject in *one* place.

A simple, hard-backed binder generally works best and takes up the least amount of space. Unless the classroom teacher has another system, each binder can be separated with a set of five tab dividers into the following sections:

- **Notes.** Ideally, students take a sheet of paper out every day to take class notes on, though this can also be done digitally (see "Virtual Binders," on page 128) and then are arranged by date. I strongly suggest that students keep their notes on loose-leaf paper rather than in spiral notebooks. In addition, five-subject spiral notebooks should be avoided if at all possible.

- **Homework.** This section eliminates the "I finished my homework but left it on the printer" problem. When a teacher gives a homework assignment, students put it in the Homework section before they complete it. After it is finished, homework is placed back in the Homework section before it is turned in. Homework is not checked off as completed until after it is back in the Homework section. With this system, homework is in only one place.

- **Handouts.** For English class, the Handout section might contain photocopied short stories, poems, or essay-writing packets. For science class, it might have lab reports or dissection illustrations. Students should remember to put the date on all handouts. It is hugely helpful when gathering materials to study for the upcoming test.

- **Quizzes/Tests.** This section is for old quizzes and tests, so students can review what they don't know and prepare for final exams. This section is also a great place to save review sheets that teachers hand out to help students prepare for exams.

- **Paper.** Reinforced binder paper is one of my favorite school supplies—it is a bit more resilient than regular binder paper. Students really need only twenty or thirty sheets of paper in this section, and can refill when necessary. As more schools are doing more assignments online and digitally, some students make the mistake of thinking they don't need any paper—inevitably, they do.

VIRTUAL BINDERS

It's late on a Sunday night, and your daughter knows she completed an assignment on the computer but forgets what she named the file. She's cranky, you're annoyed, and there are only so many documents she can open without losing her mind. What a way to start the school week!

The drive to go digital means that students and teachers need to devise a single system that incorporates both computer-accessed material and the traditional handwritten work that will always be part of what they use and produce. But keeping track across media is often cumbersome. The method I have settled on is to have students simply reproduce their physical binders digitally. On a computer, it is easy to create header folders titled Math or Social Studies, with the familiar subfolders nested inside: Notes, Homework, Handouts, and Tests/Quizzes. This way the conceptual layout is consistent; however they're accessing the material, they always know what to do, where to put that paper or file, and where to go to retrieve it.

An additional key is to have a weekly regroup time when students go through any unfiled documents—the digital equivalent of crumpled papers in the backpack—parked on the desktop or elsewhere and sort them appropriately. Otherwise, the desktop can turn into the over-stuffed backpack, and the Sunday-night search continues.

NAMING FILES

Does your daughter have computer files with clever names like "SallieHW12"? How ingenious! How easy to remember a week from now! I have worked with students to come up with a simple solution.

If your daughter uses a computer that is shared by others, her file names should include her own name as well as the subject, chapter, and date. Here's an example:

SallieBioC3RevQ111213: This file name means Sallie's biology chapter 3 homework that includes review questions and was completed on November 12, 2013. It should be placed in the virtual folder Sallie > (subfolder) School > (subfolder) Biology > (subfolder) Homework.

If your daughter has her own computer, she can forgo her own name and keep the rest:

BioC3RevQ112213: As before, this file name stands for biology, chapter 3, review questions, completed on November 22, 2013, and is saved in a similar tree of folders and subfolders.

TIP

A file notebook system like Evernote can help girls easily organize files that are then accessible from multiple locations. That way, even if she does forget to remove her homework from the home printer, she can easily print it out if she has access to a school computer. Dropbox is another tool many students use to keep their files accessible from multiple computers and avoids the annoyance of constantly emailing files to oneself.

FAQ: BINDERS

1. My child's school is a laptop school. Does she need real binders as well?

In a word, yes. Over the past few years, I have consulted with students, faculty, and parents at laptop schools who are struggling to find that ever-evasive balance of technology and technology-free. The problem is that going digital often includes the promise of being paperless, but this is almost never the case. Invariably students still receive and generate physical papers that they need to track.

So there will always need to be a balance. Perhaps, in predominately laptop environments, students will not need a binder for each subject. But I do suggest as a minimal fallback position that students retain at least one binder separated by subject, with four tabs for each subject (Notes, Homework, Handouts, Tests/Quizzes) and one Paper section at the back. This is a miniaturized version of the system described in this chapter. It would look something like this:

English—Notes, Homework, Handouts, Tests/Quizzes

Science—Notes, Homework, Handouts, Tests/Quizzes

History—Notes, Homework, Handouts, Tests/Quizzes

Math—Notes, Homework, Handouts, Tests/Quizzes

Paper section

2. My daughter's teacher has his own method for organizing binders, and he inspects them for a grade.

If this is the case, students by all means should use the teacher's method. Keeping in sync with the school or class requirements comes first. The system presented here is a workable model for those who can choose their own organizational routines. Whatever system is used, or if there is the leeway to adjust the organizational method suggested by the teacher, I always urge the prioritization of simplicity and workability. A student is most likely to keep up with a system that is reliable and consistent.

3. What about having one overall homework folder in which all assignments that need to be turned in that day are kept, regardless of the class?

Sometimes parents or teachers recommend this method. I find, however, that it's usually better to keep work for each class separate. Ultimately it's easier, when thinking about work for English class, to go to the English binder for *everything related to English class*: for storing the homework assignment, looking through past work that might be relevant, and reviewing for a test.

4. My daughter insists that chorus, health, art (or other similar subjects) do not need a binder. What do you think?

Students often tell me that certain classes, usually electives, don't need a binder, because they "don't have anything in that class." Then, of course, as we are going through their binders and backpacks, we find sheet music at the bottom of the backpack or art handouts on the Renaissance stuffed in the back of the Algebra binder. So, yes, everything needs a binder or a set and defined space—maybe a half-inch binder if there really aren't a lot of papers, but the syllabus and handouts for health need to go somewhere other than the back of the social studies binder.

5. That sounds like a lot of binders—my daughter has seven classes. How can she manage it all?

I work with a lot of students who have seven classes, and there is always a way to manage the load. Many schools have block scheduling, in which students have only a few classes each day. If that is the case, your daughter will need to carry only the three or so binders for the given day's classes. If her schedule includes all classes every day, I suggest that she use her locker between classes to store the books and binders she doesn't need (I know this does not always happen). Some schools issue double copies of textbooks, one for home and one for school, so students don't have to lug them back and forth; this also reduces the total load being carried. Even more recently, some textbooks are available digitally, which reduces the physical transport load.

6. My daughter is in junior high, does not have a locker, and one day a week she has all her classes. She cannot carry seven binders. What should we do?

I completely sympathize with this problem, which is shared by some of the junior high students I know. There are a couple of options: (1) You could get her a bigger backpack or a rolling backpack if she does not already have one. (2) If you really want to consolidate classes into one binder, first combine the electives or classes with the least paperwork: art and health, for instance, or chorus and foods class. For these smaller classes, double up a single binder: include two sets of the four dividers (Notes, Homework, Handouts, and Tests/Quizzes) and use a single Paper section at the back.

PLANNERS

Most schools give out daily planners to their students, and the majority of these go underused and can be found stuffed in the bottom of the backpack or in the desk drawer. One benefit to using the school-issued planner is that it generally lists the school schedule, with holidays or other closures. But sometimes the planner itself is badly designed; some have so little space to list homework assignments that your daughter would have to use a magnifying glass to fit everything.

If your daughter's school doesn't provide a planner or if the planner is inadequate to her needs, have her get her own. Most office supply stores have a few good options. Ideally, the planner would be at least five inches by seven inches and have ample space for homework assignments, upcoming tests and quizzes, and extracurricular classes and personal activities.

THE ALL-IN-ONE-PLACE SOLUTION

Here's something that happens all the time: A girl who seemed to have everything in place comes into my office, mid-semester, completely stressed by an out-of-control schedule. She is anxious and indecisive. The cause of the problem, as we soon discover through our conversation, is too many different organizing media. She's tracking some information in her school planner, keeping other bits on her cell phone, and admits that her mom runs a master calendar of family events at home. All of these overlap ambiguously. She never knows where to look for any one item. Her biology teacher just sprang a last-minute test and now she is *So.Stressed.Out.*

Generally, I pull out a piece of blank paper and have the student list all the different assignments, obligations, and issues she has going on and then all the tasks she has to get done. Next, we take out her planner and prioritize. She writes down homework on the night it's assigned, writes out all her different sports practices and extracurricular obligations, and schedules when she is going to do her work each night of the week. In fifteen to twenty minutes, this blizzard of half-perceived commitments is reduced to a quiet list of known scheduled items. Relief slowly starts to set in. A planner can be a very efficient brain dump that transfers all her worries from her mind to the paper, where they can be seen and considered for what they are (rather than what they were feared to be).

TIP

Have girls write down homework on the night it's assigned rather than the day it's due. This simple trick helps them learn to be proactive about doing work. If she has a big test or long-term project due in several weeks, have her start at the end and work backward: write the assignment at the top of the due date and then have her write down several reminders (and mini-assignments) to herself along the way. On Sundays, have her map out her week with all of her assignments, and block out when she is going to do homework each night. Ideally, as I describe in the next section, she sets aside a two-hour block each evening Monday through Thursday, with two to three two-hour blocks over the weekend.

THE ONLINE HOMEWORK DILEMMA

In the last few years, many schools have moved to online homework hubs. The idea is to make all assignments available to all the students (and parents) all the time. But these systems work well only when they are operated consistently, and inevitably they bring their own special problems. My experience using such systems is that, despite the promise of greater efficiency, teachers still struggle to set homework standards and students still struggle with organization and time management.

In my consultations with schools, I generally recommend that all homework for the upcoming week and any grade updates be posted on Sunday evening or Monday morning. In an ideal world, the homework would be posted by the Friday before, so those students who needed extra time or who have packed schedules would be able to work proactively over the weekend and budget their time accordingly. Everyone—students, parents, teachers—would understand that this is the only time the information will be refreshed. This puts a clear ceiling over users' expectations: They know the extent and limits of the system and can plan within it. Students in particular benefit from seeing their responsibilities clearly laid out and from having sufficient time to schedule the work to meet them. One local private school limited updates to once a week because so many students and parents were feeling increased pressure to constantly monitor the online system.

> Have girls write down homework on the night it's assigned rather than the day it's due.

I do not universally oppose posting homework online or using online systems of homework management, but I do think they should be used as a secondary rather than primary source of information. Teachers should still announce homework in class and write it on the board and should take a moment to encourage students to copy it into their personal planners. Consequently, my advice for students is simple: Use a personal planner to track all the different elements of your life and use the online system as a backup.

ELECTRONIC VERSUS PAPER PLANNERS

In the last few years, the proliferation of smartphones and other electronic devices has made keeping track of assignments digitally a more appealing option. However, as with online homework systems, the reality is usually less exciting than the idea. I have yet to encounter an electronic planning system that works really well for students, for two main reasons. First, most systems have trouble tracking long-term assignments; they make it hard to visualize progress, and keeping on top of daily assignments with long-term projects quickly becomes cumbersome. Even if daily reminders or weekly reminders are set up, they are quickly ignored. Second, most junior high and high school girls struggle with social distractions as it is and keeping assignments in a smartphone or other Internet-connected device just increases the temptation. One goal of good scheduling is to *separate* focuses; digital planners usually confound this goal for preteen and teenage girls.

Scheduling Homework and Free Time

Parents often wonder how I convince students who struggle with organization and time management to adapt this system, and I have found it to be fairly straightforward. I make it all about them. Most preteen and teenage girls would love extra free time, and understanding that adapting the system and related habits can radically decrease their stress and increase their free time can be a major motivator for making changes. Using the methods of organization and time management that I teach in my office, students regularly find that they can free up an extra four to six hours every week. That's a lot of time; over the course of a school year it can amount to over *150 extra hours* that can be used for hobbies, pursuing interests, hanging out, socializing, relaxing, or sleeping.

> I make it all about them.

My core recommendation is that students commit to setting aside two-hour blocks, Monday through Thursday, for doing homework. Ideally, this time is scheduled for as early as possible after the school day ends. A girl who may have been up since six a.m. (or earlier) and has been at school all day is already pretty tired, and nothing is more time intensive than trying to complete work when exhausted. If she comes home right after school, then four to six p.m. would be a good time slot. If she plays a sport or is involved in another after-school activity, the time block will have to fit around her practice schedule. It is important that she schedules her time herself, so she feels in control and is actively making the commitment in her mind. It's *her* work, and when she begins to assert control over her own tasks and time, it's great for her to feel the genuine satisfaction of having made a real change for the better.

Depending on a girl's age and course load, she might need to do some work over the weekends, and if that is the case, setting aside two or three two-hour blocks can work well. If she schedules the time, she will be less likely to have that gnawing anxiety that comes with unfinished work. On weekends, I always suggest that students finish all assignments *before* Sunday evening, say, before five p.m. Scheduling ahead of time, with realistic and eminently doable chunks of time, is the best antidote to the Sunday night blues. It also gives students a bit of a breather to relax before starting a new week, instead of beginning Monday morning sleep deprived.

Some schools have block scheduling in which only a few of the students' classes meet each day, and students will therefore generally have two days to complete homework. For planning purposes, simply making the shift from trying to do some homework on the night it is assigned rather than the night before it is due can make a big difference. Nothing is much worse than leaving math homework until after soccer practice on Thursday night, only to discover, already exhausted from the long week, that each of the nine problems has five subparts, so there are actually forty-five problems awaiting completion. Deciding to think and plan ahead can avoid these meltdown-inducing revelations.

PITFALLS AND STRATEGIES FOR SCHEDULING SUCCESS

The key point in constructing the homework blocks is this—*two hours of scheduled, committed attention, free of distractions, every day.* For girls, freeing themselves of distractions can be particularly difficult in an environment constantly invaded by digital bleeps, tweets, and the allure of technological communication. A conversation over text can seem efficient while doing math homework, except for the fact that forty-five minutes later she has exchanged very little more than . . .

A: Hey
B: Wht up?
A: Hmwk
B: I am so bored
A: Me too

. . . and completed three math problems with dubious results. For some, creating a "Technology Box," a physical box where phones are placed (or locked) for the duration of the study period, can be easier for girls to manage than trying to resist, minute by minute, the need to check in.

There might be days when your daughter doesn't have two hours of homework; these are good times to work ahead for upcoming exams, review difficult material, or work on projects. There might be days when she has more than two hours of work (though those days will decrease significantly the more she follows this system). Remember, most girls want more free time, want to feel less stressed, and would love a few extra hours of sleep. When they see that this method is a way to make all that happen, the intrinsic motivation can kick in.

Encourage structured breaks. Flow is good: We are often at our most productive when we get so absorbed in an activity that we lose track of time. But becoming absorbed in engrossing work can also be exhausting if it continues night after night. Especially for girls with perfectionist tendencies, it can be difficult to accept and realize that taking breaks actually decreases the total work time and feels less depleting than working straight through. I encourage students to recognize their threshold and take structured breaks before they reach the point of no return. For some, that might mean a structured fifteen-minute break for every hour of work, or a half hour for every two hours.

In any case, it is important to get up, walk around, and move eyes away from the computer screen. Girls need to figure out what amount of time works best for them, and this usually occurs by trial and error or varies depending on the situation.

FAQ: SCHEDULING

1. My daughter is in junior high. Is allotting two hours for homework appropriate?

It really depends on your daughter's classes, the expectations of her school, and how long it takes her to get work done. Schools should generally assign around ten minutes of homework per grade level, so a tenth grader ostensibly has about an hour and forty minutes of homework (I realize this is not always the case). That could vary, of course, depending on how many advanced classes your daughter is taking, or if she studies a foreign language. She also could take more time if she has learning differences that necessitate more labor-intensive study techniques. But I have found that two hours is an accurate estimate for most junior high and younger high school students. Older high school students and those taking many honors and AP classes will likely need more time.

2. My daughter cannot sit still for two hours. Suggestions?

Two hours is a guide, and students' ability to focus without distractions varies. For some students, two hours can seem like an eternity. Collaborate to find a solution—perhaps she can start with thirty or forty-five minutes of work followed by a timed ten- to fifteen-minute break. If she repeats that pattern three or four times, she will have reached the two-hour study block time. Again, this is a model for her to adapt to her own styles and preferences. (Though

I should add that it is also often useful to use two hours as a goal: Most students will need to work for this long at some point and should not be encouraged to reduce their study time simply because they aren't used to working steadily.)

3. **What if my daughter does not have two hours of homework every night?**

The two-hour block is not just for doing homework. It is also a time when students can read upcoming chapters in their science textbook, make flashcards, and complete review sheets—anything that helps them become more proactive in their schoolwork. The idea here is to have *a set* time, each day, scheduled for schoolwork. In the next chapter, I discuss long-term strategies for studying; if she has extra time on a given day, your daughter can implement some of these to get ahead, ease the burden of following days, work on a looming project, and so on. Keeping with the two-hour blocks, even on nights when they think they have only fifteen minutes of immediate work, helps students radically reduce the number of late-night cram-fests made worse by printer jams, lost files, and crashing Internet connections.

4. **My daughter has a learning difference, and even though she is fairly organized, her homework regularly takes her four to five hours without distractions. Any thoughts?**

Some of the organizational techniques can help reduce the amount of time your daughter spends completing her homework. Encourage her to take set breaks in between—perhaps a half hour for every two hours so she can get outside or do something she enjoys and finds relaxing. Our efficiency diminishes over time, so that fourth or fifth hour could be wholly unproductive because she is so tired. But the bigger-picture question is this: Why is she taking classes that give her four or five hours of homework? Are there ways she could reduce her workload if she is feeling overwhelmed?

5. It takes my daughter thirty to forty-five minutes to figure out what the homework is between texting friends and checking the online homework calendar. Does that count in the two hours?

Much like gathering ingredients doesn't count toward baking time, hunting down the homework doesn't count toward the homework time. This is one of the reasons it is important for students to keep their own record of assignments rather than relying on online or other support systems (like the phone- or text-a-friend method favored by so many). If she has trouble regularly instituting a personal planner, ask her to come up with some strategies for making keeping her own records easier.

EXERCISE

Instead of coming up with set rules, collaborate with your daughter and have her come up with ways she can be most efficient. Have her experiment to see how much time she saves if she is able to work free of technological distractions, take structured breaks, and complete homework on the night it's assigned rather than the night before it's due. You should ask her how you can be supportive, and she should tell you about what roadblocks she needs to overcome in her efforts to become more organized and efficient.

WHERE TO STUDY

During presentations in schools, when I ask students about *where* they do their homework, there is a common reaction. Usually, more than half the audience admits that they do their homework in their bedrooms. And when I then ask if they have ever spent fifteen minutes staring at the paint color on the wall or wondering if maybe they should change their wall poster, a low-grade giggle breaks out, first here or there, and then spreads across the room. Students look around at each other as if to say, *Really, you too?!*

If at all possible, the bedroom should be a place of rest. Many girls confess to doing their homework in their room, and often on their bed. This is a terrible idea for a number of reasons. First and foremost, most people's brains (I hope!) associate their bed with sleep and rest. When students attempt to be alert and attentive in their place of rest, their brain and body become confused. It can become common for parents to walk in to find their child fast asleep on her bed with books strewn around and homework unfinished. Other students rouse themselves in the wee hours of the morning to finish the work they didn't get to when they dozed off while studying. Find alternate study spaces.

> If at all possible, the bedroom should be a place of rest.

In addition to being a place for rest and relaxation, a girl's bedroom can potentially be messy. Moving out of the bedroom can be a huge and unexpected mental relief. When setting up a homework area, think about ways to control the inevitable mess; maybe placing cubbies or organizational catchalls in the dining room or office for storing materials would alleviate the sprawl of homework supplies.

I realize that in some homes, the bedroom is the only option. Perhaps there are multiple younger siblings running around or there is no dining room or other free space in your home. If that is the case, simply find a way to designate a space in the bedroom for work, preferably with a desk that is not facing the bed. If other children are the problem, consider bringing the whole family into the study period routine. Younger kids who don't have regular homework can read, draw, or play quiet games. It's never too early to promote the habit of spending some time each day in quiet mental activity (sometimes it is easier said than done, but worth a shot). Here are a few other useful tips:

- **Find several study spots.** I encourage students to come up with three different study spaces where they feel they can effectively get work done. These spaces can vary based on a girl's personal learning style and preferences. Good study spots include the dining room, especially if the space is free from technological and other distractions, and the kitchen, if it has a big table where books and materials can be laid out. Some girls might prefer to do work in complete silence, whereas others will want the comfort of having others around or background noise. Varying study spaces can help girls get ready for the future, when they may be away in college or working in an office environment and must be flexible enough to work under different conditions.

- **Library time.** Going to the library a few times a week can be a great way for girls to learn how to work in a space outside the home. It is an extremely useful habit to develop before leaving for college, where dorm-room distractions can make it impossible for even the best-intentioned student to get any work done. Many of my students make a point of going to the library once during the week and once over the weekend. Sometimes parents go along for the ride on the weekend and use the drive as a built-in collaboration period. Most girls will admit that two solid hours at the library is more effective than four hours attempting to do algebra and history homework in a messy bedroom. Older high school students might prefer to work in coffee shops or other places where there is a bit of background noise. The goal is to identify several good work spaces that work well, and have girls become flexible about rotating between several different spots.

TECHNOLOGY: FRIEND, FOE, OR BOTH?

When I talk to students I often shock them when I reveal that I am not completely opposed to the use of social networking sites. Many students are so used to being told to avoid technology or stop texting that it is a refreshing change when an adult says it can be okay. Social networking, online communication, and text messaging are this generation's way of feeling connected, just as the landline telephone was for previous generations. Indeed, our digital age provides the opportunity for girls to potentially pursue their sense of purpose and personal goals using technology. And if we want our girls to be on the cutting edge of new opportunities, they need to feel comfortable and in control of new possibilities. On the other hand, social networking needs to be managed, like everything else, and prevented from becoming a deterrent and hindering a girl's personal progress.

Remember, however, there is no doubt that many kids (and adults) struggle with low-level forms of technology addiction. Students—and adults—can have a tough time with technology self-regulation, especially when it comes to distinguishing between using technology for work and for play. The problem can be so intense that many adult writers go to the length of paying for software (such as Freedom) to block their Internet connections for a set amount of time (I simply disable my wifi connection). For students, too, the temptation can be irresistible: that ten minutes of checking Facebook turns into an hour of going through a friend's most recent status updates, music choices, and photos. Or the fifteen-minute break reading online magazine articles swells to two or three times the scheduled length. And even, for example, in a collaborative online meeting between student study partners, in the mix of checking the posting about the science project's requirements and talking about that big history presentation, conversation all too quickly drifts into other pressing topics, like Who is Rebecca's date for the dance? Did you hear that Joey got in trouble? And can you believe what happened in Mr. Slater's class? Even though that is all best left to after homework, it is becoming more and more difficult to regulate and separate work time from social time. For kids who struggle in these areas (and this is most of them), I strongly recommend the use of the previously mentioned Technology Box as a place where technological gadgets like phones go during homework and sleep time. Some students have admitted that they wished their parents enforced a Technology Box system (parents can't ever win, can they?). Students should also do all homework that requires a computer last, and turn off their online social systems.

It is also important to address how ostensibly school-related online work can easily get sidetracked. As our technology morphs and evolves, we now face nearly daily challenges to technology policy and professionalism. As schools and administrators set policies, new technological innovations sidestep the rules and create more potential land mines. Some schools now deal with the confusing phenomenon of teachers and students using social media to communicate with one another. This practice has become especially prevalent among younger teachers who are eager to incorporate familiar social networking technology for class-related work and communicating with students. While inventive efforts to engage students in learning new material should certainly be lauded, teachers must also understand that social communication with students can have the potential liability to blur the lines of teacher–student professional boundaries. I am glad to see more and more school districts coming up with set policies about teachers' use of social networking sites with their students. There is still work to be done, and this is an ongoing collaborative conversation. Teachers should generally keep their communication with students separate from their personal social networking simply as a matter of good policy, and schools should continue to set and review guidelines on appropriate methods of communication. Parents should raise concerns if something seems potentially inappropriate or otherwise confusing and should start by having an honest conversation with their daughter about good online communication.

Putting Organization into Practice

I realize, of course, that it is all well and good to provide a list of organizational tips, as I have done in this chapter. It all sounds great, when laid out on paper. But you may be wondering how to actually implement these ideas with a girl whose personal mood seems to change faster than the phases of the moon. You may see the potential benefits in these strategies, but you may fear that whatever you're suggesting will be met with eye rolling and a deep sigh.

Each girl is different, and it is hard to say in advance what will be greeted with excitement and what with skepticism. But I do know this: We all inherently want to be well rested, relaxed, and confident. We want to feel good about our abilities and find ways to make our lives easier. Girls may not want to admit that the ideas were helpful, especially if a parent is the one who introduced them. In particular, it can be helpful for girls to use such recommendations in the context of the larger effort toward focusing on purpose and fun discussed in the previous chapters.

So, with that in mind, here are some tips for implementing the suggestions:

- **Soft introductions.** The material in this chapter and the next one can be introduced in a variety of ways, depending on a girl's age and attitude. Many girls have found it helpful to first read the information in these chapters on their own. They can then meet with parents or mentors and think of solutions collaboratively. Remember, whatever works best can be the right choice, and solutions can vary with the circumstances.

- **Revisit the importance of parental attitude and approach.** If you are a parent who wants to implement these strategies with your daughter, remember the importance of parental attitude and approach discussed in Chapter 3. I realize that simply by being the parent you are sometimes at a disadvantage, because you and I could say the same thing, and your daughter would find me super helpful and you would get a look of contempt. But take a moment to reflect: What are you potentially doing or saying that could be deterring from being successful? What change could you make so that this process can be more productive?

· **Collaborative cooperation.** No one likes to be forced or told what to do, least of all a preteen or adolescent girl who is pretty sure she is smarter and/or cooler than you. Coming up with ways you can work together or side-by-side can help make this feasible. Maybe one mutually convenient Sunday afternoon at the beginning of the semester can be scheduled as a collective big regroup time, and you could go through your papers while she goes through hers. Getting organized doesn't have to be stressful or boring, and the end relief can be remarkably stress relieving. It's just getting there that can be the challenge.

· **Set a timer.** When girls want to get organized, they often feel overwhelmed by the simple act of getting started. There's so much to do! How will they know they're done? This could go on forever! A good rule of thumb is to have her set a timer for two hours and see how far she gets in that stretch. Toward the end of the two hours, have her clean everything up, set the work aside, and go do something fun (preferably outdoors if the weather is nice).

· **Weekly regroup time.** Even with the best of intentions, we all get off track. This is why so many New Year's resolutions fail; many of us are fine at making commitments, but we have trouble keeping ourselves accountable and getting back on track when challenges arise. One reason the students I work with are so successful at keeping themselves on track is that our weekly sessions serve as a built-in weekly regroup time. Maybe a girl started out the week strong, with good habits and a solid plan in place, but something happened socially with friends that made it impossible to concentrate, or she got into an argument with her parents on Wednesday night about a sleepover that upcoming weekend and everything fell apart. Resetting at the start of a new week keeps such small distractions from becoming permanently disruptive. I recommend scheduling a weekly regroup just like anything else. Sunday afternoon is a good time, when everyone can set up for the week ahead. It can be especially helpful to arrange to regroup with someone else, perhaps a parent or friend. (Special Note: If a girl spends time between two households, collaborate to make sure both homes are set up with similar standards if at all possible.)

Part of the collaborative exercise, for example, could be coming up with a set weekly time to reorganize her binders and backpack, map out her week, and pencil in appointments for pursuing interests like those in Chapter 4. Even though it would be nice if we could all instantly become more organized and purposeful and practice constant self-compassion, kindness, and empathy, we need to be realistic. Focus on progress rather than perfection, and use the weekly regrouping time to get back on track.

TIP

Regroup times can also be a good time to reflect on what worked in the previous week, what didn't, how your daughter was able to spend her time, and what she would like to change in the upcoming week.

· **Outsource as necessary.** Maybe the right person to help your daughter implement these ideas is an older mentor, an aunt, or another adult whose relationship dynamic is more conducive to this sort of thing. Perhaps it could be a cousin who is hip and cool, or a family friend who plays a mentoring role in her life.

· **Regroup at the end of the semester or school year.** At the end of the semester, your daughter can use one of the regroup times to move all physical papers that aren't immediately needed to manila folders and create a file box that is separated by subject. That way, if the papers are needed in the next grading period, they can be easily accessed, but if not, she isn't needlessly carrying them back and forth to school. If most things are stored digitally, creating virtual folders can help get them out of the way of daily stuff. Another option would be scanning the important files and filing them on the computer, a great backup system. That way, she always has the work in case the teacher's computer crashes.

A Helpful School Supply List

GENERAL

- **Binders.** 1-inch hardback binders for most subjects, ½-inch binders for smaller subjects, 1½-inch binders for classes that have a lot of paperwork. **(Note:** If your daughter is at a laptop school where most work is done on the computer, getting one or two binders, as described earlier in the chapter, is fine.)

- **Tabbed dividers.** One set of five-tab dividers for each subject.

- **Planner.** Use a page-a-day or other style that has ample room for students to write schoolwork and extracurricular activities.

- **Reinforcements.** For binder paper or handouts.

- **Reinforced binder paper.**

- **Three-hole punch.** One for the home and a portable one for your daughter's backpack.

- **Pencil pouch.** Preferably made from canvas because the plastic ones often break.

- **Calculator.** Wait to see what type your daughter needs for class.

- **Stapler, tape, scissors.** For the study space at home.

- **Markers, pens, pencils.**

- **Big erasers.** Preferably Staedtler Mars plastic eraser or something similar.

POST-SEMESTER STORAGE

- Manila folders

- File box or file system

- Graph paper

OPTIONAL

- Basic art supplies for projects

- Book of quotations

- Non-electronic dictionary and thesaurus

||||||||||||||||||||||

CHAPTER SIX

Rome Wasn't Built in a Day

Strategies for Quizzes, Tests, Projects, and Finals

Whenever I ask a school audience if they have ever been up late on a Sunday evening completing a long-term project or presentation for Monday morning, I hear a few groans and lots of nervous laughter. Whether it's an audience of squirmy sixth graders or well-heeled parents, I see the same looks of shamefaced recognition, as if to say, *"Why, yes, how did you know that was how I spent last Sunday night?"* Procrastination is not age specific. It crosses all socioeconomic and cultural boundaries, and it affects girls as well as boys.

Because it is so uncomfortable, procrastination naturally brings with it a lot of rationalizing. The majority of kids and adults who tell me that they perform better under pressure or do their best work at the last minute have rarely done work any other way. The adrenaline rush that kicks in when a project is due in less than eight hours and a person who is simultaneously hyped-up and sleep-deprived generates a kind of hallucination of productivity. Firing on all cylinders for a few-hour stretch, exhilarating as it may seem, is both deceptively inefficient and unsustainable over a long period. The following crash is often longer than the high-octane work period. And when girls fall into a pattern of depending on this kind of pressure to get their work done, they inevitably burn out, and often in more areas of their lives than simply the academic. In addition, such a work cycle can wreak havoc as they juggle hormonal changes with sleep deprivation and adolescent anxiety. This can also totally disrupt any efforts to fit new interests into a schedule because everything else gets shoved aside when the long-avoided deadline hits.

> Firing on all cylinders . . . exhilarating as it may seem, is both deceptively inefficient and unsustainable over a long period.

It doesn't have to be this way! And it is important to try to see that it is not this way, especially for girls who are trying to juggle the many different stresses in their lives.

Previewing Isn't Just for Movie Theaters

Leslie was one of my very first students. When we first met, she was a high school sophomore. She had recently been diagnosed with learning differences including dyslexia and ADD, and the educational psychologist recommended that she work with me for additional support. When we started working together, she was spending hours looking over material using strategies that didn't actually work for her. Over time, we were able to work together to find strategies that were effective and useful for *her*, which included listening to books on tape while reading along and previewing the class lessons ahead of time. She learned that being organized and proactive helped mitigate the extra time it took her to digest some of the more challenging material. When Leslie implemented these strategies, she started feeling more confident in her abilities and became engaged in her classes in ways she never had before. Her teachers frequently noted the positive difference her previewing of the material made in her class participation and performance. Instead of feeling bogged down by her academic challenges, Leslie was able to understand and own how she learned best; she then took those strategies and newfound self-knowledge into other areas of her life. Today, she puts her extreme organization and time-management skills, as well as her personable nature, into something she really enjoys—working as an event planner.

For many students, previewing the material can make a huge difference in their classroom confidence and comprehension. For students who are shy or anxious in a classroom setting, understanding what is going to be presented in class ahead of time might make them more inclined to become actively engaged and participate. For those who get distracted easily, seeing information before it is presented in class can make it easier to focus rather than wandering off at the first sight of confusion.

The Law of Diminishing Returns

When I talk with girls, we often discuss how much longer schoolwork takes when they are tired. But it is not only exhaustion that undermines their performance. It is also the habit of starting work too late or working, as a compensation for procrastination, for hours and hours without a real break.

For example, think about a project or longer-term assignment that is supposed to require approximately five hours to complete. Students have two weeks to finish; those who break the task into four or five dedicated work periods can get it done relatively painlessly. If the printer runs out of toner or the formatting isn't working as hoped somewhere along the way, it's a minor annoyance but it's not the end of the world. The student can keep going and tend to the glitch or put the whole thing aside as she gets tired and return to this later. She has this flexibility because she can always come back to it later.

Conversely, a student starting the project the night before the deadline is *counting on everything going right*. She's hoping that computer trouble won't waste half the night, that a crucial book or set of notes will be available, that she won't discover the need for some background knowledge she was supposed to learn and now doesn't have time to acquire, and so on. It's important to acknowledge the holistic nature of getting work done, even in the best conditions. Many small elements make up the possibility of productivity: physical health, adequate energy, access to the necessary resources, cooperation of technology, absence of rival demands for time, etc. Not only is the procrastinating student avoiding the discomfort of acknowledging how behind she is but she is also constructing, necessarily, a whole series of idealizations about how smoothly the late work will go. And generally, when she leaves things for the last minute, what would have otherwise been a minor annoyance becomes reason for a Grade A Meltdown.

BREAKING DOWN PROJECTS INTO MANAGEABLE PIECES

One of the reasons students experience so much stress from the amount of work required of them is that they often have a difficult time breaking bigger assignments into manageable pieces. Thinking about how to finish an enormous project is much more overwhelming than, for example, scheduling time to visit the library to do preliminary research. Using their planner, girls can take a bigger assignment and map out their strategy for getting it done by creating mini-assignments along the way. Some teachers do a great job of enforcing this in their classrooms; others leave it to the student. Sometimes, when students are left to do it on their own, they are at a loss as to how to break a project down and then avoid the task and hope the entire project will magically disappear or go away. In my office, I sometimes see that simply sitting by a student and helping her talk out the different steps can be enormously stress relieving and that the student is much more likely to break down the project if someone is there to collaborate. If that is the case, having her use her weekly regroup time to map out time lines and long-term projects can be a good use of that time.

Quizzes and Tests

Do I believe quizzes and tests are the best indicators of future performance in life, let alone future academic performance? Not necessarily. As I've mentioned, I believe that teaching to the test and the push for officially sanctioned achievement encourages a kind of learning response that is not helpful for the full development of many girls. But tests are not going away any time soon, and given that fact, it is important to figure out how to incorporate studying for them into a sane, responsible, and productive work schedule.

Some classes have a few quizzes here and there, whereas others have a daily or weekly quiz as part of the classroom structure. Girls sometimes feel so much stress about the idea of lots of quizzes that they go too far in either direction: overcompensating and doing far too much or doing far too little, trying to ignore the fact that the quizzes account for 20 percent of their overall grade (unfortunately, the pretend-it's-not-there-and-it-will-go-away strategy usually isn't as successful as we would hope). Here are a few tips for making quizzes more manageable.

READING QUIZZES

One of the most common mistakes students make is trying to cram the reading for a quiz into the night before. It may seem to be an efficient method but it actually undermines the brain's best learning. In general, we learn best when we are exposed to the same information multiple times, and we are allowed to review it. So girls can maximize their chances for retention by spreading the studying over two or three days.

Simply coming back to something they have already encountered imprints the information more lastingly into memory. It also allows girls to see exactly what they don't know and then to concentrate on repairing that, the root of most progressive learning.

Some students tell me that they like to read before going to bed and so save their reading for last. Reading before bed is fine for pleasure reading, but our mind tends to unwind and start to wander to sleep when we're comfortably situated in bed, so it's probably not the most productive way to take note of the multiple literary devices in Shakespeare's *Hamlet*. I encourage students to schedule their reading assignments into the normal block of homework time like any other task. This doesn't mean reading has to be done strictly, though—perhaps there is a comfy chair or other designated reading spot that has good light and minimal distractions.

If your daughter struggles on reading quizzes, she should look back and see why she isn't retaining the information (this assumes, of course, that she is actually doing the reading in the first place). What strategies has she tried that didn't work? What other approaches could she brainstorm for the future? If she learns better through audio processing, perhaps listening to an audio book while reading along would be useful. Or maybe writing out some simple flashcards with the essential information would help her absorb and retain the information. Here are some other tips:

• Encourage her to divide the reading up into smaller sections instead of trying to tackle it all at once, especially with dense reading. Every few pages or chapter or so, she could stop and ask herself what she thought was important and jot down a few notes. It could be plot points, characters, or questions she has about the material. The key is that she is actively engaging with the material and constructing, in effect, her own review sheet. Even if she doesn't completely understand everything, her active reading will help her ask questions and create a summary that can guide future reviewing.

• If she has several days to read the material, she should use the night before the reading quiz to go over her notes and look over the reading, instead of trying to read the material for the first time. The combination of being tired and feeling pressured to complete something breeds anxiety rather than confidence.

VOCABULARY QUIZZES

Sometimes the simplest learning methods are the most effective. Ordinary index cards, for example, are excellent tools for learning vocabulary or indeed any kind of card-size facts. There are now some great online apps that can help students create flashcards, which can be helpful especially if a student is traveling. But I still prefer the tactile approach of creating flashcards from tangible index cards: The hands-on act of writing out the words and definitions reinforces learning through another pathway. When a girl creates her own study devices, she can use all sorts of creative tricks for triggering stronger memories. Creating full sample sentences or drawing pictures are two good methods. Students who get good at this often remember their funny associations years later.

MATH QUIZZES

Students who struggle on math quizzes sometimes mistakenly believe that studying simply means staring at the material and then staring at it some more. Not so much. Instead, here are two important steps to studying for math quizzes:

• *Create a review sheet.* Her review sheet should consist of all the relevant formulas, broken down and explained in her own words. Alongside each formula, she should include a sample problem, not straight from the textbook but rather her way of explaining it to herself in numbers. She should try to assemble the review sheet in advance, so she has time to use it, put it away, and come back to it. It shouldn't be a laborious process—just a clear, direct overview in a form she easily grasps.

- *Complete sample problems.* Redoing sample problems can help calm nerves and inspire confidence. Perhaps there are old problems from class notes or homework that can help her review the material. Compiling a few problems and creating a pretest of sorts can help her see what she knows and what she tends to forget and also helps alleviate some anxieties that might creep up on test day.

MAP QUIZZES

I also recommend the pretest, flashcard approach as a way of studying for geography tests on capitals, states, and/or countries. An easy method for studying is having your daughter print out ten or so blank copies of the map she is going to be quizzed on. She can go through one of the maps and fill in as many as she can from memory. Then she can concentrate on learning what she doesn't know and repeat the exercise as many times as needed. There are now several different online geography tests; some teachers might recommend using those as well. I do recommend taking the opportunity to mimic the quiz situation as closely as possible, so if the quiz is a paper quiz, it's important to fill out at least one blank map by hand.

FOREIGN LANGUAGE QUIZZES

For most of us, learning a first language was likely a deeply sensory experience: grabbing objects and having adults name them, spelling words with blocks, feeling new pronunciations stick on the tongue. It's too bad when students study foreign languages as merely intellectual exercises. I've met some incredible language teachers who do their best to bring all five senses back into the classroom. After all, it isn't simply about conjugating verbs or memorizing the predicate.

Learning a foreign language isn't going to happen by cramming the night before a quiz. Parents can always help review new vocabulary words and terms, and the laughter elicited by bad pronunciation can actually promote better memorization. In addition to reading and writing sentences, finding ways to expand the sensory experience can further encourage comprehension. Software such as Rosetta Stone and Fluenz can also serve as supplements to traditional textbook practice.

BIG TESTS

For some students, fear of big tests can block preparing for them. They get so caught up with the idea of being overwhelmed that they waste enormous amounts of time explaining their worry rather than working to alleviate it. The best way for girls to break out of this cycle is to break down the test preparation into manageable steps.

First, she should collect all the relevant information already covered in the class. Everything she needs to know *should* be somewhere in her notes or previous work. She should gather her notes together and retrieve old tests—again, in a digital age, she might be able to have them stored on her computer. Is there a review sheet? Some teachers, especially in junior high and high school, give students specific review instructions before exams.

With all the materials gathered, she can start the process of reviewing in an active way. Over time, girls identify methods and patterns that work best for them. Some might start by outlining their own notes. For others, going through a virtual online presentation or putting together a pretest from homework and quiz questions is most helpful. Some girls crave collaborative review; for them, going over the material with a parent or a friend feels less isolated and intimidating. Simply skimming the review sheet is almost never enough; especially for a test covering an enormous amount of material, it's crucial to work ahead and put the materials together two to three days before the test date. Doing so can make the whole process of studying seem more manageable. It's not uncommon for students to get seventeen-page math review packets or history review sheets with over two hundred terms. Sitting down and trying to plow through all the information in one night can quickly become exhausting and overwhelming. Before even starting, students should decide what they think they can reasonably do in one sitting. Then they should schedule out their preparation time over several different time slots.

And, as with homework and projects, girls need to remember to allow for breaks and collaborative time. It's difficult to retain information when a brain is on virtual overload. Creating space to take regular breaks within the study routine is crucial for maximizing absorption and understanding and minimizing stress.

WHEN THE INITIAL TESTS DIDN'T GO WELL

Some girls panic when they do badly on a test or not as well as they expected. It can be difficult for some of them to acknowledge that this is only one test among many and is not a definitive judgment on their intellectual abilities and self-worth.

This kind of reaction is often exacerbated by the perception of how friends are doing or how they think their parents will react. Parents will sometimes say to me, "I know Jaime gets her biology test back today, and we're *praying* that she improves from that last test." Or the parent will go online and find out the score before Jaime can even break the news. Not helpful. It only contributes to the toxic environment in which a girl views her score as a reflection of her worth.

If your daughter has been struggling on tests, resist the urge to be reactive and upset. Try hard to show a rational and measured response. (I know that can be easier said than done.) Tone down the implied and explicit expectations and instead encourage her to use the disappointment as an opportunity to figure out how she learns best. Here are some tips:

- If she is upset, wait until she is calm, and then encourage her to look over the questions and try to figure out why her answers were wrong. She may need to enlist the help of the teacher or work with a tutor—this can be a very positive development in developing her own problem-solving strategies. Be patient. Don't assume she understands even the smallest conceptual steps. Have her work step-by-step to figure out exactly what she wasn't grasping. Many times, girls who were initially dejected by a poor test grade can actually gain new confidence from understanding where they erred. After all, understanding how we learn and knowing how to bounce back from challenges is the ultimate long-term goal.

- Encourage reflection. Use the disappointment as an opportunity to think about the approach to studying or to revising work patterns. For instance, some girls can really digest material well when working in groups and collaborating with others, whereas others need to study in complete solitude. Many people need a combination of both. Brainstorm different solutions without judgment or expectation. She can make changes by committing to making the review sheet ahead of time, working with a peer tutor on a regular basis, or going over the material aloud. Even if you think she could be working harder, having her come up with solutions is generally more effective than you telling her what solutions she should come up with, and it helps her build her own critical thinking and problem-solving skills.

- Encourage her to find different ways to experiment with learning the material. Some students tend to stick with one way of learning even when it isn't suiting them and don't inherently make the connection that there are many ways to learn material. The exercise on page 109 might promote thinking through some different options. In the long run, learning how we learn best is one of the most crucial confidence-building life skills.

Girls implicitly want to do well and feel good about their future and possibilities. We all do. If academic performance becomes too alienating, girls may start looking for other ways to find satisfaction. This may result in engaging in detrimental compensatory behaviors (see Chapter 8) to numb the pain from frustration and angst. If they continue to struggle academically, encouraging girls to be their own best advocate and speak with their teacher and school counselor might be a good place to start.

TESTING ANXIETY

Imagine feeling devastating dread every time there is a math quiz or test. Now, imagine there are math quizzes or tests at least twice a week and anxiety bubbles over until the results get returned, which are almost always demoralizing anyway. Girls can put such enormous pressure on themselves that they can almost feel the physical weight of the real or imagined expectations of those around them. Some can quickly turn relatively minor academic happenings into catastrophes. I regularly see girls who work themselves into a frenzy thinking that if this one test doesn't go well, they will never get into the honors class next year, and then no college will admit them, and then they will never get a job, and then . . . the panic itself then becomes an impediment to problem solving and action-oriented learning. For some girls, defusing the fear can be a first step toward resetting a vision of their life so they can begin to take ownership of their learning process.

Testing anxiety is real. The high-stakes world of testing in both public and private schools across America has left many girls (and boys) with an underlying anxiety about taking tests. Children as young as three years old are instructed to fill in bubbles and compete for correctness; some are told that their future success depends on each right answer. It might seem that with all these different tests and because testing now begins so young, that most students would build up a kind of immunity to test anxiety. But curiously, more and more students struggle with testing anxiety and related panic. Restlessness, sleeplessness, loss of appetite, nervousness, nausea, headaches, profuse sweating, shortness of breath, and dread are all real symptoms that can dramatically affect test performance and overall mental and emotional wellness. Some students begin to avoid school and regularly become sick on test days, and others become so fidgety and nervous that their mind goes blank in a testing situation.

Many girls are ashamed of their fears, which they come to regard as a strange lack of self-control. Some girls admit that their parents' (real or imagined) expectations can contribute to or exacerbate their testing anxiety. These girls typically do not realize that panic attacks in relation to tests (or sometimes even to class participation) are real and fairly common, and that there are specific strategies for dealing with them. Left unaddressed, such fear can build up and overflow into other aspects of their lives. It is much better to encourage an environment in which girls feel comfortable articulating their concerns without the fear of consequences. Here are some strategies that might help:

- **Re-create the testing scenario.** For some students, re-creating the testing scenario beforehand and taking a practice test at home a few nights before the classroom test can be helpful in envisaging a better outcome. This strategy can be especially successful for students taking standardized tests. In our office, students who re-create the testing scenario report feeling more confident on the day of the test because they know what to expect. Even more important, they learn not to be afraid of their own responses to a stressful situation and to work through to find solutions.

- **Maximize sleep and relaxation before tests.** Work with your daughter to devise a relaxing night-before-the-test routine. Maybe she will take a twenty-minute bath before flipping flashcards and heading off to bed early. Perhaps one of her methods will be to avoid technology the night before exams to screen out potential social-networking drama. Remember, it's not just the sleep the night before the test—which can often be disrupted by nerves—but the sleep quality for several nights before a test that can affect our overall alertness.

- **Be mindful of morning routines.** How a girl starts the day can also impact her ability to concentrate on her math test in fourth period. Collaborate to come up with some strategies that work for her. Maybe certain breakfast foods and a cup of tea might offer comfort. Perhaps having all her materials and backpack set out the night before helps her become more relaxed on the morning of the exam. Even knowing what outfit she will wear in advance might help.

- **Visualize.** Visualization works. A few nights before, the night before, or the morning of an exam, encourage your daughter to take a few moments and visualize the quiz or test going really well. Ask her to explain (to herself or others) how that would look and feel so she can mentally practice being calm in the testing situation.

- **Thirty seconds, five deep breaths.** When the teacher hands out the test, I recommend that students take thirty seconds to take a few deep breaths and become refocused and relaxed. During the test, if they feel anxiety rising, repeating this strategy can get them to take a mini time-out and get back on track.

- **Take a break.** Sometimes, during an actual test, despite the best preventative techniques and efforts, students feel the anxiety creeping in and start to panic. For some, getting up and taking a break can be a good technique of last resort. I realize that some teachers have classroom rules that may impede being able to get up and walk around during the test. Talking to the teacher beforehand about the possible need for such action can make it easier to feel comfortable doing it in the middle of the test, or provide alternatives that could also be helpful. Or the teacher may be able to come up with some alternatives that fit within the classroom structure.

- **Seek support.** If your daughter keeps struggling with testing anxiety, encourage her to talk with her teacher or school counselor. A supportive adult might offer some classroom strategies or extra advice that could make a difference. Talking to a psychologist or therapist might also be helpful in developing individualized coping skills and dealing with deep-set fears.

Long-Term Group Projects

Just the mention of the phrase *long-term group project* evokes groans from students and distaste from even the most supportive parents. Perhaps you are remembering when your daughter's group left her with the bulk of the work and you found yourself racing to the art-supply store late Sunday night to find some necessary but obscure tool for a three-dimensional diorama. Or maybe the group members were meeting at the house farthest from yours at a time that meant you hit traffic both ways. However, if girls go into long-term group projects incorporating some of the interests piqued by material in earlier chapters, these projects can potentially be fun and fulfilling. And these projects can become highly practical for students' eventual post-school lives. Ultimately, out in the real world, most of us need to figure out how to work collaboratively regardless of our career choice. We likely interact with individuals whose personalities and work habits will differ from ours, and a key element to finding personal success is learning how to work through those differences to find a bit of harmony. So when your daughter complains about a long-term group project or the people she has to work with, listen with empathy and ask her how she can proactively work to make the situation better for everyone involved. Here are some tips to help make projects a positive experience:

- **Think before joining.** I realize that sometimes students aren't given a choice, but when they do get to choose, friends don't always make the best group members. Looking outside the immediate social circle can actually be beneficial. If your daughter has a bad group experience, have her take some time to analyze the problems after the dust has settled but before another project begins. What could have been done differently? What lessons can be carried forward to future projects? Perhaps she was too accommodating in letting everyone dump tasks on her. How can she be assertive and also polite in making sure she isn't being taken advantage of? How could the delegation of tasks be handled more fairly? Brainstorm and collaborate to encourage her to come up with solutions. These are not simple matters with simple solutions—part of the point of working in groups is learning to negotiate in situations where she doesn't have complete control. These are all extremely useful life skills, both for school and after.

- **Break the project into smaller tasks.** If project management is not included in the assignment, students can work together to map out and track progress on a long-term project. Maybe using a shared online spreadsheet (for example in Google Docs) or some other program can help everyone understand the delegation of tasks.

Have your daughter schedule the individual pieces in her planner, timing everything so that the last bit is done a day or two before the actual due date. Creating an extra block of time on the weekend before the due date—but not on Sunday night—can avert the night-before-it's-due-broken-printer scenario.

- **Take advantage of helpful technology.** There are many ways to arrange group video chats using free online applications. Having the meetings online can potentially actually reduce the hours typically wasted at someone's house "working on a group project." Of course, the group chat cannot cover experiential work, like filming a video, but it can be quite useful for delegating tasks, creating presentations, or practicing parts. As always with technology, a certain level of maturity and focus are required, so depending on her age, you may want to have her complete online group conversations somewhere that you can keep an eye or an ear on things.

- **Encourage your daughter to incorporate her interests.** In Chapter 4, I talked about identifying areas of personal interest and enjoyment. If she can incorporate such interests into school projects, it may be another opportunity to see if that interest could be something she would like to actively pursue. Say, for example, one of her interests is learning how to produce videos, and the project offers an option of developing a video presentation. She may feel more comfortable writing a traditional essay—but a more interest-enhancing choice could be a great chance to enhance and expand her abilities.

- **Think progress, not perfection.** If your daughter has trouble with group members or is trying to work through something and you know there is an easier way, let her figure it out or talk through some of the challenges. Resist the urge to insert yourself into the process and take the lead. Be a background voice, a listening ear, and a source of advice when it's asked for. Letting her work through the natural rough spots of collaboration is to allow her to really learn from the process.

Final Exams

More than anything, Stephanie dreaded those few weeks each year when finals seemed to loom large. Her shoulders would begin to slump and her eyes would hollow in dreaded anticipation. She turned both focused and distractible as she made to-do lists over and over in her head. Though she generally seemed reserved and in control, Stephanie's internal anxiety spilled over and found loud expression in seemingly unrelated areas. She would have a mini-meltdown when her mom forgot to buy her favorite breakfast cereal or when her brother left his math homework on his desk and they had to run back home and were late for school. Finals invoked a fear in Stephanie that she couldn't verbalize or completely comprehend, but if she had been in the Department of Homeland Security, those few weeks would have been permanent Code Red.

Part of the problem was that Stephanie had created an enormously complex system of routines in order to prepare for finals. The core of these routines was mostly a series of time-intensive and laborious processes that didn't really help her actually understand and absorb the material. She spent hours and days perfecting minuscule tasks and methods that left her exhausted but no closer to her goal of understanding the material and feeling ready for the set of upcoming exams. When finals finally arrived, she had done both too much and too little, and her results were often disappointing to her.

FINALS STUDY SCHEDULE

In my office, I have a simple, streamlined system for preparing for finals that I have used for more than a decade. Former students who are now in college regularly tell me they use the same system to study for their university exams. It is all about the principles I have emphasized throughout this chapter: breaking down the studying into manageable parts, rotating between exam subjects to avoid burnout and exhaustion, and taking regular breaks.

Here's the plan:

1. **Create an exam packet for each subject.** About a week before finals, your daughter should gather any final review sheets, important notes, old quizzes and tests that are relevant to the material to be covered. For each subject, she should create a packet filled with all that information. The idea is that if she went to the library with nothing but the packet and the course textbook, she would have everything needed to study for the final. I do realize that many of these review documents can now be easily scanned and stored digitally, but my experience is that many students find it easier to use a tangible paper that can be flipped through, written on, revised, and ultimately mastered.

2. **Create a finals study schedule.** Using the Finals Study Schedule Form on page 170, have your student break up her time into a series of two-hour blocks. Each block has slots for two subjects: She can rotate within that time block as needed. All the work of studying, both organizing material and reading through notes, is done in the allotted periods. The goal is to complete the prep work—assembling any and all review sheets and constructing all flashcards and supporting materials—at least two days before finals start. That way she avoids the trap of overemphasizing preparation and deemphasizing review, and the days immediately before the

169

Finals Study Schedule Form

WEEK BEFORE FINALS

	Monday	Tuesday	Wednesday
Afternoon 3–5			
Evening 5–7			
Evening 7–9			

FINALS WEEK

	Monday	Tuesday	Wednesday
Morning 10–noon			
Afternoon 1–3			
Evening 4–6			
Evening 7–9			

1. Put together a manila folder or envelope packet for each class. The packet should contain important notes, homework assignments, old tests and quizzes, and the final review sheet.

2. Make flashcards or do practice problems for *everything* on the review sheet.

3. Finish all review sheets, practice problems, and flashcards by
_____ (date).

Thursday	Friday	Saturday	Sunday

Thursday	Friday	Saturday	Sunday

exams are spent reviewing and mastering the information rather than making flashcards or filling out study guides.

3. **Exercise, sleep, and nutrition.** I talk more about the importance of exercise, sleep, and nutrition in Chapter 9, but for now let me simply emphasize that they are all central to exam success. It seems logical but is often overlooked. Girls who go through finals week don't inherently make the connection that they cannot perform at their peak sleep deprived and stressed out. Most people understand that they shouldn't stay up all night or eat junk food before running a marathon, and yet some girls regularly do both before final exams. Ensuring that students get adequate sleep and make better food choices in the week before exams makes an enormous difference in the way they feel. Students who follow the schedule and complete their review sheets ahead of time are more confident and calm about their overall finals experience and feel much less anxious and overwhelmed. It is not surprising that they also do well on the actual exams.

> Most people understand that they shouldn't stay up all night or eat junk food before running a marathon, and yet some girls regularly do both before final exams.

||||||||||||||||||||||

CHAPTER SEVEN

Social Wellness

Putting the Fun Back into Fun and Games

Less than five minutes into my meeting with Kelly, I knew that something was amiss. After I gently asked her if anything had happened in school that day, she started trembling and then the full tears and uncontrollable sobbing burst through. Between gulps, she explained how a girl in her class had texted their entire group of friends, telling them to go to a different event from the one Kelly was performing in later that week. This girl and Kelly had a long competitive friendship—that is, they were seemingly friends but more like frenemies.

The incident had completely derailed Kelly's school day; she couldn't concentrate on anything else, including working on the English essay she was trying to revise. After identifying the problem *as* a problem (not always easy for girls who are actively participating in a damaging relationship), we discussed strategies for dealing with her classmate, particularly how to disengage from a toxic relationship in a way that is empowering. Easier said than done, but simply being conscious about having the choice to curb or end relationships can be enlightening.

Middle school and high school can be a great place, or an awful place—and for some girls, it just depends on the day or week. Girls are in the challenging position of trying to juggle their evolving relationships with their friends and potential romantic interests as well as their parents and other adult authority figures. The notion of fitting in and being socially acceptable can be of utmost importance to some girls, and their judgments can be clouded by their overwhelming desire to feel accepted and liked. Girls who feel ostracized can easily resort to detrimental behaviors to compensate for the pain caused by the isolation, especially if they lack the coping skills to deal with their own individualized reality. One of the key steps in social wellness for girls is to help them develop self-awareness and break free of the compromises they make to fit in.

> One of the key steps in social wellness for girls is to help them develop self-awareness and break free of the compromises they make to fit in.

When I ask girls what they like to do for fun, a common refrain is, "Hanging out with friends." For many girls, hanging out with friends can be relaxing; after all, having supportive friendships is incredibly important for our own sense of personal wellness. At the same time, though, most teenage girls find that friends can also be a source of drama and stress; many girls knowingly recognize their friends and/or frenemies are sources of both joy and pain. There are two real risks here: One, that girls who are funneled into social-media-driven friendships don't have time to be "off" to reflect, process, and learn from their different experiences. The other is that girls, under the encroaching influence of these entertainment and technology-driven styles of friendship, fail to develop the skills that lead to supportive, lasting, spirit-enhancing relationships. These are what I call *real relationships* because they are supportive, are authentic, and come from the interests of the girl herself rather than from the preprogrammed image of friendship that she imports from outside.

Character formation is of special importance during this crucial time of development for girls. I don't mean to imply that there is any single or simple image of what having good character looks like. Defining character can be massively variable across individuals, families, and cultures. Regardless of that, we all want our girls to develop and espouse the attitudes and characteristics that underlie genuine, authentic relationships. Unfortunately, we know that, especially during socially stressful adolescence, that is often not the case.

In my work, I see how comparison and judgment are at the root of most girls' social ills, especially as they relate to socioeducational struggles. Female social relationships have always been complex, but there now seems to be this unwavering and deep-seated meanness and instability that is starting younger and younger. Our schools and society create an environment in which comparison and competition are commonplace and, in many cases, ultimately detrimental. As Brené Brown notes in her book *The Gifts of Imperfection*, "Comparison is all about conformity and competition. At first, it seems like conforming and competing are mutually exclusive, but they're not. When we compare, we want to see who or what is the best out of a specific collection of alike things."[1] Indeed, today girls can go online 24/7 and view someone else's edited life through Facebook, Tumblr, Pinterest or blog postings, and the subconscious (or conscious) comparison and competition can lead them to wonder how all those people are having so much fun or leading such great lives. These profiles highlight the irony of trying to pursue real friendships in the somewhat fake world of cyberspace; when everyone has a carefully self-selected online persona, it's hard to know what is actually real. Psychologists today work with adults who have a hard time distinguishing their online profiles from real-life persona, and this same phenomenon can also affect preteen and teenage girls. The online social world also adds another layer of competition and comparison and can make it even more difficult for girls to learn to feel comfortable with their own state of being. And, once a girl starts comparing herself to others, she is susceptible to forgetting about what her interests, abilities, and talents are in favor of how she matches up to her friends and peers.

Comparison then leads to judgment and contempt and is a way that girls (and many adults) rationalize their vulnerabilities by feeding off of the insecurities of others. If a girl feels bad about herself, she can reason that it's okay because another girl is so much fatter/uglier/stupider/poorer than she is. And with judgment often comes the eye-rolling and exclusionary tactics of relational aggression that have become frighteningly commonplace among girls.

The epidemic of girls' meanness is one result of this confusion of values. When girls are mean, they diminish themselves by acting in a way that gives them temporary relief from the personal emptiness they may be experiencing. They often have a hard time acknowledging how their values may be in conflict with their actions, or they have never stopped to truly develop their own set of personal values. When girls are taught to identify and to value the elements of real relationships and mutual friendships, they can learn how to create conditions of their own social happiness. A girl who is secure in her friendships and, above all, is confident in the priorities she places on being a good friend and seeking positive friendships that are in accord with her own acknowledged values becomes more immune to the self-emptying behaviors that tempt many teenagers.

In our hypercompetitive and ever-changing world, developing good communication and collaboration skills can take the backseat to cutthroat rivalry and vindictive behavior. A girl's friendships and relationships can quickly shift; her best friend could betray her trust and ignore her when a new group of friends shows interest, and the boy who smiled at her in the hallways and texted every night could now be paying more attention to the girl who sits next to him in math class. Even friends who are outwardly supportive of one another can have an underlying competitiveness. The drama associated with constantly shifting social dynamics and hierarchies can leave even the most confident girl feeling frayed, and the resulting anxiety can have her turning to box-filling behaviors to assuage that uneasiness. As neuropsychiatrist Louann Brezendine notes in her book *The Female Brain*, the teenage girl years can be succinctly described as "drama, drama, drama."[2]

Reality Show and Cele-bratty Relationships

In recent years, girls are exposed to more and more negative models of friendship. Look at any reality show or teenage docudrama: back-stabbing, vindictiveness, and betrayal are common and somewhat expected behaviors. Are these media influences establishing new norms for future generations or are they merely mimicking what already exists? I would argue that it is a little bit of both.

In the upside-down world of reality television, it is good sport to watch grown women systematically betray the fake friendships they set up for the sole purpose of being betrayed. We can say that these shows are excessively dramatic and even that they follow a formulaic script that highlights a mere sliver to how girls socially interact within their own lives. In actuality, these shows reflect the complex workings of emotional maturity that girls have always been adept at turning to their advantage. This is a very basic driver of the boxed-in dilemma. And as Kelly's story from the beginning of the chapter suggests, toxic versions of these interactions can be more influential and commonplace than we would like to think.

The question then becomes, What do these shows and related media present to girls as an acceptable way of treating others and of treating themselves?

One of the most popular and enduring reality series, *The Bachelor*, pits young women against each other for the affection of one man. As the female contestants are rejected one by one, they invariably question their self-worth, and wonder aloud about what they did wrong. Many reality shows, including *Jersey Shore* and *Keeping Up with the*

Kardashians, popularize the phenomenon of the microcelebrity—the idea that being famous just for being famous is in and of itself a worthy goal. More often than not, the women on these shows can behave in a way that is rude, vindictive, and full of narcissistic drama. Even though those women are, for the most part, in their early twenties, many of the viewers are younger and are still forming their own values and developing their own interpersonal skills. Having such stark and dramatic examples on television gives concern for what has become the new normal of acceptable behavior.

One of the most important first steps in promoting social wellness is recognizing and understanding all the forces that combine to influence and challenge girls' social development. Though it might be easy to think that your daughter doesn't watch those shows, and as parents you limit their television watching ability, websites and online streaming options make it easy for girls to access what was once deemed as off-limits. Indeed, the many different ways of watching television shows have "actually led to an *increase* in total TV consumption from 3:51 to 4:29 per day."[3] And even if your daughter doesn't watch such shows, chances are that her peers do, which gives you every reason to share concern and want to be informed about the messages that these shows convey. It is important, now more than ever, for parents and adult educators to be aware of the messages that the media send to our girls and how that translates to classroom and schoolyard behavior.

EXERCISE

If your daughter watches television, what shows does she watch? Do you know? Watch a few television shows with her and have a conversation about what messages those shows send and how realistic they are in relation to your daughter's life. Does she know girls who behave like the ones on the shows? What shows are her peers watching? Which reality or television shows are popular with

her cohort of friends? Even if you know what was popular last year
or even six months ago, chances are there is something new being
talked about.

Virtual Relationships

Modern teenagers spend countless hours per day using their computers,
camera phones, and related social technologies to communicate with
one another. According to a 2011 Pew Report titled "Teens, Kindness
and Cruelty on Social Network Sites," 95 percent of teenagers aged
twelve to seventeen use the Internet, with 70 percent of teenagers saying that they go online daily. In 2011, nearly 80 percent of teenagers in
that age range used social networking sites such as Facebook or
MySpace, up from just 55 percent in 2006.[4] For some, the Internet and
social networking sites seem to provide an easier medium to initiate and
develop friendships, and there are now ever more ways to meet people
and to keep in touch and to do so more and more extensively. For
some teenagers, online opportunities can be comforting and positive—
teenagers who are sick and unable to attend school or are dealing with
sexual identity issues, for example, might find a supportive online network that brings them solace. And we should not underestimate the
positive impact that social media can have in helping students become
more engaged in connecting with causes they care about. In 2012, Julia
Bluhm, a fourteen-year-old eighth grader from Waterville, Maine,
started an online petition on Change.org to protest *Seventeen* magazine's airbrushed depiction of teenage girls. Within months, her petition had gathered over eighty thousand online signatures, bolstered by
postings on Twitter and Facebook and garnering intense media cover-
age. In the August 2012 issue, *Seventeen* magazine editor in chief Ann
Shoket drafted a "Body Peace Treaty" in response to the outcry and
vowed to make significant changes and become more transparent about

the magazine's photo policy in its active effort to "celebrate every kind of beauty."[5] Social media has tremendous power for good when used resourcefully, and the potential of girls' use of social media should not be undervalued or underestimated.

However, this also means that a bigger proportion of young people's relationships are devoid of face-to-face communication, which can lead to increased misunderstandings and underdeveloped social skills. For teenagers who are still sorting out their friendships and personal values, online communication can create another layer of complication. Technological communication provides a false sense of intimacy because individuals interact in a less vulnerable state. Many teenage girls can hide behind this veil to say or do things they wouldn't feel comfortable saying or doing in person. Technological communication can also convey a false sense of belonging; in following the status updates and making comments on other people's posts, girls may think they know someone when in actuality they are merely privy to the edited or online version of the person's personality.

The situation is compounded and made urgent by the enormous popularity of virtual communication. The fear of missing out keeps some girls online and connected even when they are within the physical presence of people they want to be connecting with. *Who could be texting me in the thirty minutes that my phone is in my backpack? What life-altering status update or wall posting could be happening when I am not logged in?* Lunch breaks or social gatherings are punctuated by pauses during which everyone at the table checks their technological device to see if anything earth-shattering has transpired in the ten or so minutes they were having a conversation. Who among us has not seen teenagers use their technological devices to connect with others virtually rather than have a face-to-face conversation with the person sitting next to them? This phenomenon is clearly not exclusive to teenagers; more than a few adults are guilty of the same practice.

So girls seem to build big, rich social worlds, but they are then proportionately more liable to be upset by status postings, events that they are not invited to, and other people's relationships. A girl can become unglued after seeing friends' pictures and status postings about an event she wasn't invited to, and subsequently realize that she is no longer included as part of the group she once thought she belonged to. More than a few girls have realized that the guy they were talking to is now in a relationship with someone else, highlighted by photos or relationship status changes. The sort of mean manipulation that has always been present in some girls' relationships is now much more public and more permanent. Things tend to linger in cyberspace, and reputations online can stick damagingly to their real-life subjects, even when based on misinformation and malicious truth. Increasingly, schools are having to deal with the fallout from online postings and spreading of rumors as well as the choices girls make to post photos and videos of themselves and others.

"AM I PRETTY?"

On YouTube, young girls who look to be in junior high post anonymous videos of themselves asking viewers to leave comments on whether they are attractive. In their homemade videos, these girls look desperate in their pleas, and some pointedly ask the viewers to be honest, assuring the audience that they can handle the truth. Some comments are positive but many of the anonymous comments posted are demoralizing and degrading. In one case, a mother was surprised to be contacted by local television personnel after her daughter had posted a YouTube video titled *Am I Pretty?* online.[6] Though it is common for girls this age to seek the acceptance of others, it would be safe to assume that most girls seeking the input of the World Wide Web on their physical attractiveness might be dealing with some level of insecurity. And although the age minimum for YouTube and Facebook is currently thirteen years old, who is to say that even a thirteen-year-old is socially and emotionally ready to handle the onslaught of anonymous public opinion?

It's easy to believe that your daughter doesn't really use the computer or that you monitor her interactions with vigilance or that you trust her choices. Instead of focusing on an endless battle to control access, parents need to stay informed and understand how to use the technology their kids are using. For parents, becoming informed of the different features on social websites and figuring out the different ways to use technological gadgets is a first step. What was popular three or four years ago may now be obsolete. For instance, iPhone and Android phones have capabilities that many parents are completely unaware of and that teenagers use for a variety of purposes. Parents should have full ability to monitor how a phone or computer is being used. It doesn't necessarily mean that parents should sneak around and steal their daughter's phone whenever it is released from her death grip, but rather that there is a clear understanding that full access to the phone will be invoked if you think that she is doing something harmful to herself or others.

> Instead of focusing on an endless battle to control access, parents need to stay informed and understand how to use the technology their kids are using.

It should be noted that there is an entire burgeoning industry around monitoring children's online behavior. Parents can secretly set up systems to track texts, email, and other virtual activities. Parents can check in to see where their child is based on the location of the child's phone (think "find my iPhone" becomes "find my teenager") and see if they really did make it to their friend's house or are somewhere else altogether. This software can quickly become altogether too invasive; figuring out a balance is important so that children's safety and self-awareness are the top priorities.[7]

‖‖‖

EXERCISE

Have your daughter write down the top ten websites she visits on a daily basis. Have her give you a tutorial on how she uses the different features on those websites or different apps on her phone and talk through the ways she has seen friends or acquaintances do or say inappropriate things online to others. If she doesn't have any examples of inappropriate online behavior, do a search on articles and find a few to discuss; a quick search on "online bullying" and "teenage girls" can pull up some current events.

‖‖

PICTURES WORTH A THOUSAND WORDS

A few years ago at a local high school, several boys compiled an electronic folder of nude or seminude photos of female students. The girls had taken the photos on their camera phones and sent them to different boys, some of whom they were in a relationship with at the time but that had since ended.

Unbeknownst to the girls, these boys had combined the different images, making a personalized *Playboy* of sorts. The folder was emailed around as an attachment, and the teenage boys didn't realize that sending the attachment through their school email network would give the school administration full access to their poor judgment. In this case, the school decided to punish the boys and the girls, the girls for taking and sending the photos, and the boys for exploiting them.

Most of these girls believed that their photos would remain private and may not have realized that a photo could be distributed to a virtually infinite audience within seconds. It is easy to say that these girls were naive or stupid or trusting, but who among us hasn't done something that was socially questionable in our early teens? The difference is that now some of these mistakes leave traces that linger longer and can be distributed much more widely than in the past.

Students are often in control of technology before they have the maturity to understand the long-term impact of some of their choices. In recent years, the number of cases similar to the photo incident just mentioned has proliferated seemingly exponentially as younger and younger students have camera phones. The technological distribution of nude photos of minors can have social implications as well as legal ones. *Sexting*, the term used to describe the practice of sending or receiving explicit images over the Internet has become more commonplace among teens than many parents realize. Researchers at the University of Texas also note that it can be indicative of actual sexual behavior. In a longitudinal study of high school students published in 2012, 28 percent of teens reported having been asked to send a naked picture of themselves through text or email, with 31 percent admitting to having asked someone else for a sext.[8] Nearly all of the girls who had been asked to send a sext were at least a little bothered by the request, and girls who sexted were shown to be more likely to engage in risky sexual behaviors than those who didn't.[9] School administrators and law enforcement are now being forced to address the problem of sexting. Distribution of sexually explicit material over the Internet is punishable as child pornography in some states, and the sender of such images may be labeled a child sex offender. In September 2011, New York State signed the Cyber Crime Youth Rescue Act into law, allowing law enforcement officials the option to allow teenagers to complete an eight-hour education course in exchange for having criminal sexting charges dropped.[10] The course is designed to be an educational alternative to being charged with a crime that can have lifelong ramifications.

EXERCISE

What are the school rules and local laws in your jurisdiction about teen sexting? Before your daughter is given a smartphone or any phone or computer with camera access have her research the laws about sexting and find stories on how sexting has affected teens. Discuss and then create a list of appropriate uses of the phone and other related technologies as well as what uses will result in your suspending her access to the phone.

Female Bullying: Cyberbullying and Otherwise

When Amie started the seventh grade, her junior high school brought together students from five different elementary schools. Though she had some friends from elementary school, Amie was easily influenced by whomever she was hanging out with, and the constant state of flux in her new environment made her anxious. When she went online after school, some girls who barely talked to her at school would chat with her over the Internet. One afternoon, Nelly, a newer friend that she had met in the first few weeks of school, started chatting with her and asking her whether or not she liked Samantha, a well-known seventh grader who had the tendency to be loud, obnoxious, and mean. Amie gave her honest opinion—not knowing that Nelly and Samantha were sitting right next to each other on the other side of the computer conversation laughing the whole time.

Pretty soon, Amie received an onslaught of taunts about how her "outfits were questionable," was asked in front of a large group whether she remembered to shower that morning, and was told her hair might look better if she didn't have dead things growing from it. She received text messages saying the world would be better off without her. Amie also started to be the victim of some malicious gossip and rumors, and pretty soon other girls were scared to even be associated with her. When she walked up to a group of girls whom she thought she was friendly with, they would all turn their backs away from her and actively ignore her. When she sat down at a lunch table, the other girls who were already seated would either get up and leave or say, "We are having a private conversation, could you *please* leave?" Facebook postings on her wall would include things like "We missed you at the party yesterday!" referring to an event she wasn't invited to.

Girls' meanness has been around since long before the Internet. But now, virtual and online interactions take relational aggression—talking behind one another's backs, exclusionary tactics, eye rolling, and spreading rumors—to a much more potent and widespread level. Instead of being confined to math class or the lunch tables, such aggression can follow girls home via electronic messages, and demoralizing rumors and photos can be sent within seconds. For a victim of relational aggression, it can feel as though there is no safe place or time-out from the unbridled meanness. Research shows that 22 percent of girls in grades nine to twelve have been a victim of bullying on school property (versus 18.2 percent of boys), and 22 percent of girls admit to being bullied electronically (versus 10.8 percent of boys).[11] Although bullying on school property and electronically remains consistent for girls, it is interesting to note that the incidence of boys being bullied electronically is less than half of what it is for girls. It seems to be a much more girl-related problem.

In recent years, legislation has been introduced to formally prosecute those involved with bullying because several teen suicides have made parents and administrators more aware of the detrimental impacts of these aggressive relational tactics.[12] In research studies on aggressive behavior, girls admitted that they participated in such behavior to alleviate boredom and to feel part of a group.[13] There are some excellent resources out there that are beyond the scope of this book, but the deep-seated meanness and active pursuit of another's misery indicates just how much today's girls feel that they are never good enough and how girls are desperate to find ways to assuage that internal emptiness, which includes turning on others deemed to be weaker and more vulnerable. In some cases, girls don't even know that what they are doing could be seen as bullying, because they don't understand and haven't had the conversations that help them make the connections between their potential values and behavior.

If a girl is actively engaged and feeling purposeful, it is not necessary to compromise her sense of self for the quick fix of self-satisfaction that comes from vindictiveness. To give both the aggressors and victims adequate social skills and understanding to move beyond such behaviors, we need to encourage girls to develop their own sense of personal purpose and self-worth. One of the ways to do that is to encourage the conscious development of personal values and real relationships.

EXERCISE

Look for recent news articles on relational aggression or girl bullying, and start the conversation about how those articles relate (or don't) to what happens at your daughter's school. Has she seen similar things happen (to herself or others)? Has she ever behaved in a way that could be considered relational aggression? How would she want to react if she saw someone else acting as a bully? Who could she turn to if she needed support? What are her school's policy and your home policy on dealing with relational aggression and bullying?

SLEEPOVER TOXICITY

In her controversial bestseller *Battle Hymn of the Tiger Mother*, Yale professor and self-professed Tiger Mother Amy Chua reveals her distaste for many common childhood rites of passage, including sleepovers.[14] Although she and I have many opposing viewpoints on child development and related issues, I must admit that on the subject of sleepovers we are in agreement (but likely for different reasons).

Sleepovers can be one of the most insidiously undermining obstacles to social wellness among girls today. First and foremost, the vast majority of sleepovers lack an essential element—sleep. Generally speaking, it's impossible, even with the best intentions, to have sound and restful sleep with friends, social networking devices, and the potential for late-night trouble so readily available. The late-night conversations, dares, and other sleep-deprived activities that typically happen at sleepovers usually result in crankiness, irritability, and annoyance in the days that follow. Even though sleepovers are in person, much of the virtual manipulations can create unnecessary drama for days and weeks to come.

I can generally sense a difference whenever a girl comes into my office after being at (or hosting) a sleepover. Much of the allure of being at a sleepover is the fear of missing out, and even girls who recognize the toxicity don't always feel confident in saying no to sleepovers. Staying at a friend's house until *right before* going to sleep can provide the social outlet without the sleep deprivation. I recommend this alternative. If, for whatever reason, you are hosting a sleepover for your daughter and her friends, I encourage one simple rule: All phones and other technological devices must be turned over for the duration of the sleepover. Let girls focus on hanging out with one another rather than creating drama via text, phone, or other social networking ways. Board games, anyone?

Distracted Relationships

One of the most challenging aspects of tween and teenage girl life is how many different challenges they encounter and deal with on a regular basis. A girl who doesn't know how to deal with a challenge, or doesn't want to, can quickly hide behind distracted relationships. These relationships provide a diversion that lets her ignore or avoid dealing with issues that may be crucial to her long-term development of self-awareness and personal purpose.

THE INDISPENSABLE CLIQUE

Nearly every junior high and high school has some version of the attached-at-the-hip, doesn't-complete-sentences-without-group-think clique—a group so entrenched in one another's lives that they are unable to do or say anything without validation or consultation with one another. Sometimes, these groups come up with names for themselves, like the Fab Five or the Sexy Six or something altogether original. Although the need for belonging is at an all-time high during adolescence and feeling part of a group can be comforting, these enclosed friendships, to which few others are allowed access, can be stifling socially. The girls see themselves as an enclosed unit, and their union distracts them from building a diverse community of friendships and relationships. In some cases, these girls speak for one another, and there is usually an underlying power dynamic within the group. The girls may let other friendships fall away and focus solely on activities that are of interest to the entire group, rather than developing their own sense of self. If and when a fallout occurs, the results can be ever so much more painful.

ROMANTIC RELATIONSHIPS

Look at any teenage magazine cover or young adult book, television show, or movie, and a potential or actual male–female romantic relationship generally plays a central role. Websites focusing on teen girls regularly dole out dubious love and relationship advice. In one particularly painful example, *Seventeen* magazine featured thirty-five ways to be a better flirt; one tip encourages girls to:

> **Ask him out "by accident."** Text him "What r u up to tonite?"
> When he replies, say, "Sorry that was for a friend—but yeah, what r
> u doing?" The tiny diss will make him work harder.[15]

The expectation, built into the narrative structure of almost all popular media, is that girls are in their most proper or desirable state when they have a romantic interest or are in pursuit of one. Girls can spend so much time focusing on a romantic relationship, either a potential or actual relationship itself, that it can become a distraction from dealing with other issues they may not know how to deal with or that may be intimidating to them.

Over the years, I have seen this story play out time and again with girls who become completely enveloped by a potential love interest. Having a significant other assumes priority above any other dreams, interests, or objectives. If and when an actual relationship develops, it snowballs into something that becomes an unhealthy and unbalanced distraction. Friendships become secondary, and the girl spends hours each evening and weekend chatting and texting with the romantic interest or analyzing their interactions in minutiae. After the breakup, the girl holds on and maintains communication in such a way that it becomes a distraction from being able to move on and foster new relationships (romantic or otherwise). For a girl who uses a romantic relationship as a distraction, the time and energy spent focused on the relationship keeps her from exploring and developing her own sense of purpose and self-awareness.

In no way am I saying that all teenage romantic relationships are negative distractions. Indeed, an important part of the developmental process is learning how to communicate and collaborate within the context of healthy social and romantic relationships. But in a world in which girls are given the message that being in a relationship actualizes and validates their worthiness in some basic way, they can easily use a romantic relationship as a distraction from their own personal growth and wellness. Think about the girl who spends all her time with her boyfriend and lets her friendships fall by the wayside or the one who, in the midst of the college application process, becomes intimidated by the thought of moving far from home and uses the fear of losing her significant other to distract herself from dealing with anxieties about homesickness and the upcoming life changes.

Real Relationships

Like everyone else, most girls long for a sense of connection and belonging. We all hope to find friends who appreciate us, who are supportive, loyal, and kind, and listen without contempt, comparison, or judgment. Most girls recognize that the friends who can help them laugh when they are having a bad day or provide empathy without judgment are the ones whom they are extra lucky to have. Though friendships change and evolve with time and circumstance, girls want the connection, support, and comfort that genuine, authentic relationships bring. As a part of building their worlds, girls need to feel empowered to realize their abilities in proactively promoting their own social wellness.

Where do girls learn how to be a good friend or how to seek out real relationships? Where do they learn the qualities that make up a good friend and what virtues are important for living a meaningful life? Sometimes these qualities get talked about in elementary school, but as girls get older, learning how to be a good friend and what characteristics and what traits to look for in a good friend often get overlooked in favor of focusing on superficial traits or artificial similarities. Promoting conscious behavior and awareness of choices in actions and words may seem simple, but it is often overlooked today. In their own cocoon of developmental self-absorption (the "me" phase) girls sometimes have a tough

> Though friendships change and evolve with time and circumstance, girls want the connection, support, and comfort that genuine, authentic relationships bring.

time looking beyond the intimate bubble that includes what impacts them and their world. We make the assumption that girls know how to deal with real friendship and relationship issues, when in actuality, reality show relationships and virtual communication styles make the development of real relationships more challenging and confusing than ever before. Instead of proactively seeking out friendships that are positive and empowering, girls can find themselves stuck in the swampland of reacting to what gets thrown at them—on the playground, in the hallways, and online.

THE JUST KIDDING SYNDROME

I was recently talking with a high school English teacher about the evolving nature of girls' friendships, and she reflected on how she can always tell which girls are friends with one another based on what they say to one another's face versus behind their backs. "There is a group of girls who are friends in one of my junior year English classes who regularly say things to each other like, 'I can't believe how *ugly* your face is,'" she explained. "And they will all break out in laughter. I know these girls think it's funny, but I know that at least one of them is seriously struggling with body self-image and confidence." Who needs enemies when your girlfriends tell you that you're ugly?

More than ever, sincerity and genuine kindness have been replaced with sarcasm and other communication styles that are more painful than uplifting.

Girls who supposedly like each other are so mean to one another, but why? When I ask the girls I work with, they admit to making similar comments. One girl proclaimed, "If your friend is eating three slices of pizza, you might kid around and say something like, 'Hey Fatty!' *but only if she's not fat at all.*" If your friends joke around that you are fat, it's not long before you actually believe it, no matter how confident you are in your body image. Cue in body dysmorphia.

Most adults could not imagine being friends with someone who told us we were ugly or stupid. More than ever, sincerity and genuine kindness have been replaced with sarcasm and other communication styles that are more painful than uplifting. It is what I like to call the *just kidding syndrome*. When something really mean and demoralizing is said with a "Just kidding!" or "JK!" that doesn't really negate what was said or how feelings were hurt, but the recipient is supposed to take it as a joke. When I bring up the just kidding syndrome with girls, they almost unanimously agree how hurtful certain joking comments can be.

EXERCISE

Asking your daughter to become more conscious of how she communicates is a first step. Ask her to keep track of comments that are either sarcastic and/or made with a "just kidding!" at the end for a full week, either in school or among friends. Reflect on these statements. If the JK were removed, how would the comment make someone feel? How would it make *her* feel?

CURB THE TECHNOLOGY ADDICTION

Young girls and adolescents today cannot remember a world without computers, the Internet, and cell phones. While most adults can vaguely recall a time where they relied on their landline and snail mail, these latest generations have been ensconced in technology from birth. This can explain why for so many it is so hard to disconnect, in addition to the fact that at this stage in development girls tend to be less able to control their impulsiveness. So even if they wanted to limit their constant checking of their phone or email or texts, it seems almost impossible. In many cases, girls actually need support with regulation and structure from the outside. For some girls, the technological addiction reaches a further level of compulsiveness; its enormous time drain provides a distraction from dealing with pressing challenges.

Several parents whose daughters I work with noted their girls' reactions when their phones were unavailable—the phone was either broken or lost or it was taken away for some disciplinary reason. Initially, the girls were grouchy, irritable, and generally awful to be around, quite like someone going through some sort of withdrawal. Once they got over that initial hump, though, the girls seemed calmer, more relaxed, and in better moods. They found other ways to occupy their time, and reveled in how much more free time they had. The girls interacted with friends in person and even came out of their rooms more often.

Most girls could benefit from a forced technology sabbatical or at the very least, a break from their phone. Maybe you devise a rule for when you are on vacation or have a basket to collect phones when other girls come to your house to hang out. Perhaps you proclaim three to five hours a week to be designated as technology-free time in your home. In doing so, you encourage girls to start thinking in full sentences and communicating in person with less punctuated intervals. Girls who took a forced leave of absence from their phones were freed to be reflective in a way that seemed impossible before. And when the sabbatical was over, many of the girls were less reliant on their phones.

CHARACTER DEVELOPMENT ISN'T JUST FOR SCREENPLAYS

What are the qualities that make a supportive friend? How does one become a loving and compassionate person? How can one develop high integrity? How are those traits developed? Are they inherent or learned? Or both?

When many adults reflect on their upbringing, they may reflect how their character was influenced—either positively or negatively—by their parents and other important adults in their lives. Perhaps the teachers and mentors who were active participants in their lives played a role. Maybe even their peers were influential in this way.

Girls today have a thousand different sources impinging on their character development. Reality shows, celebrities, and media sources all tell them how they should behave and what counts as looking and being good. But ultimately, the people who have the most lasting influence are those with whom they spend the most time or with whom they have tangible interactions. Parents and teachers and other adult role models can actually have a larger influence on character development than we are led to believe, and yet we often overlook that aspect of their roles.

EXERCISE

Sit down with your daughter and write out answers to these three questions:

☐ What do you think are the most influential components on a person's character?
☐ Who or what factors are important in building a person's character?
☐ What does it mean to be ethical?

Compare and discuss about your answers. Start the conversation about what builds good character and what you each think the important qualities are to being a person of character. You may be surprised by your student's insights and your resulting conversation.

KNOWING WHO YOU ARE AND WHAT
YOU'RE LOOKING FOR

In the race to multiply virtual relationships, girls can quickly find themselves spending time chasing quantity over quality (that is, "How many Facebook friends do you have?"). But they should be encouraged and inspired to understand what friendship characteristics are important to them and to focus on developing relationships that are in line with their personal values. For many girls and young women, this could naturally occur as they mature. In preschool and elementary school, friendships can be formed based on convenience; maybe their moms are friends or perhaps they are on the same swim team or go to the playground at the same time. Starting around the fifth or sixth grade (and in some cases even younger), girls' friendships become more defined and change based on interests and personal compatibility. In high school, designation and separation can occur once again based on interests and maturity level. But even for younger girls, certain core characteristics are clearly valuable, particularly as these counter what we all recognize as the tide of conventional superficiality. When I asked girls from different backgrounds about what characteristics made up a good friend, I kept hearing the same thing—that *loyalty* trumped all other qualities. It made me a little curious; loyalty is certainly important, but what are the other qualities that made up a good friend?

As we would continue the conversations, girls would come up with different traits, such as being a good listener, being fun, or having similar interests, but naming or understanding those traits certainly did not come easily. It made me realize that we rarely ask girls (or adults) to step back and reflect on what they look for in friendships and, conversely, what qualities and characteristics they believe *they* possess that make them a good friend to others. It seems simple, but consciously analyzing what girls are looking for in friends rather than simply reacting to whatever comes their way can make a big difference when girls are in the midst of friendship struggles.

EXERCISE

Ask your daughter, and ask yourself: What character traits make up a good friend? Come up with five or ten qualities that you believe are essential. Now have her look at that list and do a self-inventory. Do the people she hangs out with possess these qualities? Have her write down an example or two of how she exhibits those qualities. Which of those qualities does she think that she possesses? Are there qualities on that list that she would like to develop further in herself?

THERE ARE SO MANY DIFFERENT WAYS TO BE SOCIAL

When Anthea started her freshman year at a private high school, she struggled to develop friendships and to fit in. She didn't know many of the other students to begin with, and her nervous personality and lack of social sophistication made her easily overlooked in the crowd. It wasn't long before she became anxious about her lack of friends and acquaintances. Anthea felt alone and began to dread going to school. Lunchtime was the worst; the charged social scene of trying to find people to sit with was so unbearable that she began to construct elaborate avoidance routines. She would quickly wolf down her bagged lunch in the bathroom and then spend the rest of the period in the library working on homework or studying for tests. She was an avid soccer player, and she was quite good, so her parents hoped that when the winter season started she would find friends on the team. When that didn't happen, her parents became worried. Their normally cheerful daughter was starting to turn sullen and lonesome, and they could see how her changed demeanor was affecting every aspect of her life. In the course of investigating other social outlets, they heard about a local youth group from other parents they were friends with, and encouraged Anthea to try it out a few times to see what she thought. There were freshmen from several different high schools at this youth group, and it gave Anthea a fresh start and a new environment in which to interact with other students her age.

Over the next four years, Anthea's youth group became an integral part of her life. She became a group leader and collaborated with the other leaders to organize events and retreats. The experience with the youth group gave her the confidence to bear and increasingly to enjoy her school's social scene. She ended up becoming more involved in school, eventually even being voted senior class secretary. She developed more peripheral friendships and found a group of friends to eat lunch with and was friendly with a wide group of classmates. Despite all this, Anthea's youth group remained her main outlet for socializing, and she admitted that her closest friendships had grown from that experience.

Some girls feel ostracized from the school social experience, and finding friends or experiences out of school can be the saving grace that makes the school more bearable. Some girls may find their closest friends in their third grade classroom, whereas others could develop their closest relationships through shared nonacademic activities or personal pursuits. Encouraging different ways for girls to be social allows them to explore multiple avenues to experience friendship and relationship building. As relationships tend to ebb and flow over time, each of the different avenues could combine to create a complex and colorful kaleidoscope, providing nurturing opportunities for growth and development.

EXERCISE

Have your daughter create a relationship web, writing down all of her various friendships and where they began. There could be a different shape for school, immediate family, extended family, and the soccer team or acting troupe and different ways to recognize all the different relationships. You can do the same for yourself. The purpose is to help girls realize that even if one social experience isn't working out or is challenging, there are two or three others that might offer alternatives. For instance, if friendships at school aren't going well, maybe the friends at the karate studio are the ones that she can count on.

HELPING GIRLS FIND THEIR NICHE OR CARVE ONE FOR THEMSELVES

In the 1986 classic teenage movie *Pretty in Pink*, Molly Ringwald's character, Andie, is a girl who lives alone with her unemployed father in a ramshackle house. She develops a relationship with Blane, a wealthy, popular guy in her class who asks her to the senior prom. A few weeks before the prom, he backs out and uses the excuse that he asked someone else because he can't stand up to his friends. Though Andie is devastated, she decides to show up anyway without a date. In a classic line of self-assertion, Andie proclaims, "I just want to *let them* know that they didn't *break me*."

One of the most challenging areas of insecurity and deep analysis for girls (and indeed, for many women) is the development of romantic relationships. For some girls, junior high and high school can be punctuated by whether they get asked to the dance and the seeming rejection from not getting asked can be the Worst.Thing.Ever. It has become doubly complicated by the casualness of romantic relationships and how the hook-up-and-hang-out-culture has left many girls and boys wondering what actually constitutes a relationship. Girls who don't have a date for a dance or are single are left thinking, like the contestants on *The Bachelor*, that they are not worthy of love or not attractive enough or good enough in some way. Certainly in our ever-evolving world, girls do ask boys to dances—sometimes. In my office, I frequently see girls waiting on pins and needles hoping to be asked to the dance or prom, whereas most boys wait until virtually the last minute to go about finding a date. Though this is a bit of an exaggerated generalization and exaggeration, most girls want to know three weeks in advance, and most boys think that two or three days is a good amount of time for everything, including prom. If you think I am wrong, look at the number of boys (and men) swarming at the last minute to get a hold of a tuxedo for any black-tie event.

This book is all about encouraging girls to create their own world within their individualized reality. Even if their life doesn't meet up to an externally set standard ideal of perfection, girls can realize an expansive number of opportunities exist when they work to carve an appropriate niche for themselves. Even if a girl isn't an actress in a play, there are a million different ways to be involved in the play's production: writing, designing and building sets, making costumes, doing hair and makeup, and contributing to the music or lighting. The same goes with social opportunities; there are so many ways to get involved in the social scene. A girl can still be actively involved in social activities regardless of whether she has a date to the dance; she could help with the production, decoration, publicity, and night-of operations. Instead of simply sitting at home (which is a viable option for those who choose it), girls can feel more empowered by generating a new alternative that reflects who they truly are, whether that alternative means going with a friend, being involved in the behind-the-scenes production, or participating in something different altogether. Help your daughter define herself on her own terms rather than be defined by feeling that she does not belong.

||||||||||||||||||||||

CHAPTER EIGHT

Emotional Wellness
Compensating and Problem Solving

Shooters is a bar/dance club in Durham, North Carolina, near the Duke University campus. It has long been a late-night destination for area college-age students. The huge warehouse of a space houses a large bar, a mechanical bull, dance floor, pool tables, and an upstairs lounging area where lurkers can take in all the action. The country-themed establishment even installed one fake bar merely to facilitate elevated dancing *Coyote Ugly* style; no bartenders actually serve drinks from that bar, but interested parties can take turns climbing into a cage to dance above the action below. Karen Owen, the 2010 Duke graduate who gained notoriety after her forty-two-slide PowerPoint "thesis" extensively detailing her sexual encounters with college athletes went viral, mentions Shooters throughout her presentation as a place where she meets, flirts, or interacts with nearly all of the thirteen young men she ranks in her report.[1]

One Saturday night in the spring of 2012, I visited Shooters to do some field research and see one element of the late-night college social scene firsthand. I had been to Shooters only once or twice when I was a college student, and I was surprised it still existed. In fact, when I mentioned my plan in passing to a school administrator, she quickly countered that I "was a brave soul." When I walked into the place, I immediately noticed the garbage cans selectively placed around the floor to catch the rainwater leaking through the roof.

By one a.m., Shooters was packed with college students and area locals in varying states of extreme intoxication, many of whom would likely not remember all the evening's details the next day. The dance floor was primarily made up of girls who moved around slowly and self-consciously, clutching their purses with intent. A few couples paraded around the dance floor with moves that could have easily been mistaken for adult entertainment if a few articles of clothing were removed. For the most part, the boys were comfortably dressed in khaki shorts or pants, flip-flops or sneakers, and a button-down or polo shirt. They wore pretty much the same attire they might wear to class. The girls, on the other hand, were dressed in a distinctive uniform of as little clothing as possible, with skirts that could have doubled as bandeau tops and tops that looked more like swimwear. Some of them could have easily been stopped for solicitation if they had been standing on a street corner a few blocks up the street. On this chilly evening worthy of a jacket, these girls wore a going-out uniform of micro skirts, low tops, and flip-flops or platform heels.

What struck me most, though, is that very few of the girls looked like they were actually having fun. Instead, for the most part, these girls looked uneasy (and nearly naked). Many of the same girls spent their weekdays studying complex economic strategies and writing papers comparing different political theories. Gaining admission to Duke is no easy feat; in 2012, there were over thirty-one thousand applicants, and the admissions rate hovered around 11 percent.[2] These Duke undergraduates had clearly excelled academically to gain admission to such a competitive institution. These girls, however, seemed far from self-assured and looked uncomfortable while trying desperately to appear cool and social.

This scene is by no means exclusive to Duke University, and I am not trying to single out the school or their students. And indeed, there are certainly more social options than simply going to Shooters-type establishments. However, when describing this scene to a colleague, he quickly opined, "You've basically described the social scene at nearly every college campus across America."

What are some of the contributors to the excessive drinking, clothing optional, casual hookup culture that pervades many of our college campuses? Why are girls engaging in behavior that can be physically and emotionally harmful? The seeds for these detrimental and often demoralizing behaviors aren't planted in college; they start several years before, when girls learn to get through the day with different compensatory behaviors.

When girls have a problem, they can either engage in active problem-solving behavior or passive compensatory behavior. Detrimental behaviors include drug and alcohol abuse, caffeine, overeating, extreme exercise, self-mutilation, and Internet addiction—basically anything that diverts attention from the actual problem. It can also include cliques, hanging out with the wrong crowd, and unfulfilling sexual relationships. Many adults engage in similar avoidance behavior instead of actively addressing challenges in positive ways; this is not a phenomenon unique to girls. However, because girls are being faced with more challenging problems earlier, as a result of the age compression and precocious puberty mentioned in earlier chapters, they are often confronted with problems before they have ever had a chance to consider creating a network of solutions. As a result, girls become accustomed to reacting to problems rather than actively working to find solutions.

A common example is that of a girl who is exhausted because she stays up late finishing homework and being social via e-chatting and text messaging. She is silently anxious about the troubles she has with her overwhelming course load and where she fits in with the ever-changing social scene. Consequently, to assuage her anxiety by monitoring its sources, she continually plugs herself into some form of technological communication; she is on all the time. Because school starts early, she gets out of bed exhausted and sleep deprived. Instead of actively seeking out and thinking through solutions that would enable her to get to sleep earlier, she compensates for her exhaustion by drinking extreme amounts of caffeine. The lattes and energy drinks leave her fidgety, restless, and anxious. She becomes irritable without a caffeine fix and drinks more later in the afternoon to try to focus so she can finish her assignments; the caffeine then disrupts her sleep quality. Late in the afternoon and evening, because she is more tired, it actually takes her longer to get the same amount of work done than if she had used the extra time to sleep. It's a vicious, self-feeding circle.

How could she have actively tried to find solutions for her exhaustion? Well, she could have learned organization and time-management strategies to help her get her homework done more efficiently. She could have instituted an electronics curfew to promote a better sleep routine, worked with her parents or counselor to scale back her school schedule, sought out a tutor for a troubling class, and revamped her schedule so she was able to do more of her homework when she was most alert. She could have made sure that she avoided technological distractions when she did her homework, and tried to complete her homework outside of her room so she had less temptation to lie down on her bed (and fall asleep). She could have worked on her nutrition to promote more refueling so she wasn't so depleted and in need of a caffeine fix. Perhaps she needed to reach out and get some outside support from a teacher, parent, or counselor. Whatever the source of help, this prototypical girl needed some larger perspective to halt the spiral of damaging behaviors.

Girls can easily fall into the trap of devaluing themselves by compensating rather than addressing a problem. It can be as straightforward as a girl overeating when she feels sad or stressed instead of finding positive ways to address the stress (taking a bath, listening to music, spending time outdoors, engaging in a relaxing activity). Over time, what was once a little problem can morph into so much more, and girls continue to hide the root problem and turn to doing things that palliate their anxieties.

Going back to those girls at Shooters who seemed uncomfortably intoxicated: There are strong correlations between college alcohol abuse and depression and anxiety. Studies haven't necessarily determined whether the drinking contributes to the depression or the depression contributes to the drinking, but the link exists. Alcohol is, after all, a depressant. So a girl who is suffering from depression could binge drink to try to temporarily make herself forget her problems and feel better. The drinking can lower her inhibitions and quell her anxiety, and she might end up hooking up and having sex with guys she might not have considered if she were sober. Those casual sexual experiences can end up harming her reputation and sense of self-worth, which could then, cyclically, exacerbate her depression.

The statistics on teenage female mental health and emotional issues are startling. The Centers for Disease Control and Prevention reported in 2011 that over one third of high school–aged girls (35.9 percent) reported having a period of at least two weeks of feeling sad or hopeless within twelve months of the survey and reported having given up some normal activities because of those feelings.[3] Girls are nearly twice as likely as boys to suffer from depression.[4] Nearly one in every five high school girls (19.3 percent) seriously considered committing suicide, with 9.8 percent of girls attempting suicide one or more times.[5] To compensate for some of these painful emotions, girls can resort to detrimental behaviors such as binge drinking, drug use, self-mutilation, and eating issues. Nearly one in five high school girls (19.8 percent) admit to having five or more alcoholic drinks within a few hours on one given day, and an identical percentage of girls (19.8 percent) admits to self-medicating by taking drugs such as OxyContin, Percocet, Vicodin, codeine, Adderall, Ritalin, or Xanax without a doctor's prescription. And even though research studies have yet to reveal definitive statistics, self-mutilation, or cutting, has become more and more commonplace among girls trying to find a way that "provides instant, though temporary, relief from stress."[6] These girls tend to cut in areas that can be easily hidden from friends and family members, such as arms, wrists, legs and ankles.

Many cutters admit that it is a way to "feel something, even if it is pain." In other words, these girls feel so empty internally that they painfully mutilate themselves in an attempt to feel *something*.

Much of the time, the mental breakdowns and significant emotional challenges we see in girls are grounded in things that happened much earlier on and were never addressed or healed. Encouraging girls to develop good communication and coping skills enables them to seek solutions rather than hide, accommodate, and pretend everything is all right. Instead of merely focusing on the detrimental behaviors, we need to help girls put systems into place for themselves to help them actively take a stance in addressing problems rather than passively avoiding them.

It's All Okay, Except When It Isn't

It can be daunting to understand girls because they can be so skilled at hiding what is *really* bothering them; at times, trying to figure out what is really upsetting girls can be downright baffling. Many girls feel pressured, as one high school sophomore girl explained, to pretend like "everything is perfect on the outside, even when it's all a nightmare on the inside." How many times have you thought that your daughter was upset about something only to realize that her annoyance and irritation was a result of something different altogether? During adolescence, girls face the conflicting struggle of trying to establish their own identity and become self-sufficient and independent from their parents with the potential angst, agitation, and hormonal swings that can envelop them. It's natural for girls going through puberty and adolescence to want to develop their sense of self away from the parental watch, but it also means that they don't necessarily know where or how to find support when they are working through some of the most common emotional challenges surrounding friendships, relationships, school performance, and personal expectations. It is often not until destructive behaviors are discovered that the deeper emotional issues begin to be identified. There are some key signs that could be potential red flags and warrant at the very least a conversation and more likely outside help or support:

- Change in eating habits (too little or too much food)

- Change in sleep habits (too little or too much sleep)

- Crying sporadically or often

- Difficulty concentrating

- Loss of interest in things, general apathy

- Change in personality, including a big-time increase in irritability

Some girls do well, and sometimes extraordinarily well, in school as a secondary effect of the internal struggles they are sorting through. Their extraordinary academic achievement can in fact be a *symptom* of their emotional challenges; sounds confusing, right? In this age of constant competitiveness, some girls turn to academic and extracurricular achievement to secure themselves when they feel other things are spinning out of control. Other girls can see their academic performance be thwarted as a result of their social ills, and yet others feel demoralized by their academic performance and try to compensate in other ways.

On the other end of the spectrum from hiding are girls who overshare and reveal their problems in a way that becomes a desperate cry for attention and can bring a burden to their teenage friendships. If they have been diagnosed with a mental or emotional health issue, oversharers wear it as a sort of badge of honor and use it as an umbrella of identification. On the first day of one of my workshops, I asked the girls to go around the room and say their name and share their favorite food. Instead of answering the innocuous questions, one of the girls openly announced, without any prompting, that she saw a psychiatrist weekly, was diagnosed with depression and anxiety, used to cut herself, and took sleeping pills for her insomnia. As the weeks went on, it became apparent that Sara used her diagnosis to define herself. Far from being too secretive, she struck me as dangerously open. How would she feel in a few years when all of her classmates, following her own lead, had identified her as her diagnosis? Learning discretion and when and how to identify and share details appropriately is just as important, if not more important, as knowing where and when to seek help when needed.

One of the fundamental aspects of emotional wellness is to understand the importance of genuine, authentic communication and problem-solving skills. Many girls struggle to learn how to appropriately and effectively communicate their needs and can't always discern what should be shared with whom and where and how discretion should be used. Blogging and social media have blurred the lines of what is and is not appropriate communication because many young girls can mistakenly feel a sense of intimacy when behind the computer and put their personal information out there for the world to see. They are desperate to find a way to properly communicate their feelings and frustration and don't necessarily know how to do so.

Learning to Seek Support

One of the most important things girls need to learn how to do is actively problem solve and seek solutions, especially when they are in unfamiliar territory (which happens a lot in the ever-changing world of junior high and high school). The solutions need to be unique and individualized, just as each girl is different and her personality is unique.

Think about a girl who really wants to do well in school. Every semester she starts out with fresh hopes: She decorates her binders, buys new school supplies, and gets her mother to buy her favorite snacks, all in anticipation that this year will be different from those in the past. For the first two weeks, everything is fine. She turns in assignments and does well on the introductory quizzes. This is it, she thinks, I'm going to ace this semester. By the third week, though, things get more difficult and different assignments start piling up. She wants to stay on track but doesn't know how to study or how to organize herself and manage her time. Soon, she is staying up late, trying to study but not knowing how to really learn the material and starts failing tests and feeling worthless about her academic abilities. No matter how much effort she perceives that she is putting in, her dismal academic results start to weigh her down. Before long, she starts falling into the usual mix of compensatory behaviors, maybe she starts staying up late and drinking loads of coffee to try to assuage her exhaustion. Or perhaps she gives up on her classes and starts hanging around kids who don't care about school. She could easily start drinking and partying as a way to numb the disappointment.

Instead of starting down the road of demoralizing behaviors, this same girl could have sought out the help of the school counselor or found a tutor to help her learn how to study. She could have gone in after school to see a teacher who could help her go through her failed tests to figure out what mistakes she was making and try to find different strategies for understanding the material. The key to making the better rather than the worse choices is thinking and planning ahead, before an upset of any size hits. Trying to figure out a catastrophe on the fly is just as difficult as trying to complete a big academic assignment in one sitting. The results are generally not pretty. Both need to be broken down into manageable pieces and then tackled objectively rather than reacted to passively.

The C's of Success

The statistics on girls' mental and emotional health issues are startling, and the signs of concern are appearing at younger and younger ages. At the same time, the competing and scrutinizing is also starting at younger and younger ages. The connection is no coincidence.

Emotional bankruptcy is the term I use to describe the emptiness that results from being exhausted and unfulfilled from all the competing, chasing, and box-filling behavior. If we think of emotional wellness as a bank with deposits and withdrawals, fulfilling personal pursuits that promote a personal sense of purpose can be seen as deposits. Things that are done based on others' expectations or external gratification are withdrawals. At some point, when the withdrawals far exceed the deposits, we reach emotional bankruptcy, and the internal feeling of emptiness contributes to the mental and emotional health issues we see with many preteen and adolescent girls.

Parents, educators, and other mentors need to help girls fill a toolbox with ways to make deposits to promote their emotional wellness, which can be a way to help them support positive ways of dealing with behavior. The C's of Success reflect some of the qualities that aren't always necessarily directly developed in the classroom but are crucial for healthy emotional wellness and personal development.

COMPASSION

Think about the conversations that happen on the school grounds at break and lunch. Girls lament about how little sleep they got, how much they are doing, and how stressed-out they are. Very rarely do you hear a girl say, "You know, my schedule was really overwhelming, so I rearranged my obligations and cut back on some of my activities and am now able to do my work at a reasonable hour, take a bath before bed, and spend time on things that I find personally meaningful."

We frequently tell girls to be nice to others, but it's much less common for girls to understand and recognize how important it is that they are nice to themselves. Of course, it's one thing to tell girls to be compassionate to themselves, and quite another to get them to do it; many times girls don't have a clue as to how they can practice self-compassion. Realizing that just because they *can* do something (take five AP classes while playing two varsity sports and dealing with their parents divorce) doesn't necessarily mean that they *should* is something that takes time and requires active effort and reflection. Given the messages that are sent by the media, schools, parents, and peers, it can be difficult for girls to realize that taking a break doesn't mean that they are giving up. Indeed, self-compassion often takes great courage because it can mean going against the achievement, box-filling grain.

Girls who can't give themselves a break are far less likely to develop the skills to understand a differing perspective or be thoughtful to those who may be struggling in some way. And even girls who are thoughtful and kind toward others can easily be swallowed up by our arms race to get more, achieve more, and accomplish more in less time if they are unable to practice self-compassion.

What are ways girls can practice self-compassion? In my experience, it comes down to three main strategies—*play, care,* and *sleep.*

PLAY

When girls play, they are really going through task-oriented problem solving. When a young girl plays house or even a simple board game with her friends, she goes through endless opportunities to practice negotiation, compromise, and active communication. Play is such a cornerstone of healthy learning and development, and more and more studies reveal how crucial active play is to positive health outcomes.

And yet, many girls stop playing far too soon. The current challenges of age compression and higher standards I've mentioned earlier are squeezing out the play so important for healthy personal learning and development. As a result, girls are effectively robbed of their ability to develop problem-solving, negotiation, communication, and interpersonal skills within a safe environment before they face more pressing problems in their own lives.

CARE

A key component of self-compassion is self-care, yet we don't emphasize it enough with young girls and adolescents. Examples of self-care include writing in a journal, taking a bath, exercising, yoga, or another activity that brings a sense of calm and joy. It can also include taking care of how you look physically—your hair, makeup, and appearance. I hesitated to add this because it is a bit of a double-edge sword because age compression has made it seem as though third graders should be wearing makeup. But the idea of girls taking care of themselves so they *feel* good and not so others think they *look* good is key. Self-care is not necessarily primping, though feeling good about how you look and taking care of yourself are related.

Note: Until girls are able to fully internalize and understand self-care, parents usually need to help them set healthy boundaries. I often hear parents say: "Oh, Marla doesn't like downtime; she likes to be busy" when in reality, Marla is overworking herself to near burnout.

SLEEP

When it comes to emotional wellness, sleep is essential. It's no accident that every single psychiatric mood disorder co-occurs with sleep problems.[7] There is more evidence, though it is still in the preliminary stages, that sleep deprivation can contribute to the occurrence of mood disorders. Matt Walker, a leading sleep researcher at University of California, Berkeley, looks at the relationship between sleep and emotional processing. When people are sleep deprived, their brains go into an incendiary situation—"all gas pedal, no brakes," as Walker likes to say.

Studies show that key emotional centers of the brain become hyperactive and disconnected from the most rational parts of the brain when it is sleep deprived. In this state, the prefrontal cortex that deals with rational thinking is underused, which is not a good state to be in for anyone, but especially for teenagers who are already going through an intense emotional period simply by virtue of being a teenager.

Teenagers are constantly trying to work everything out; they are brainstorming with themselves and through social media to analyze and try to figure out their identity and their place in the world. A lot of that time is spent examining and attempting to process information (What did he mean? Why did she look at me that way?). Their efforts can lead to sleep deprivation as girls stay up late to talk, text, and e-chat their way to an answer. But, it is crucial to emphasize, sleep shouldn't be seen as taking away from the processing. *Sleep can actually help with the emotional processing.* It tends to have a palliative effect as it allows us to detox and debrief our emotional experiences.

> Sleep can actually help with the emotional processing.

EXERCISE

Have your daughter make a list of the different ways she can practice self-compassion. Split a page into three sections, labeled play, care, and sleep. Under each of the different headings, have her come up with three to five ways she could promote each component of self-compassion.

COOPERATIVE COLLABORATION

It's no coincidence that the level of meanness and bullying has proliferated with increasing competition for grades, scores, friends, and activities. As anxiety about getting into honors classes, private high school, and college increases, the collaboration of group projects is overshadowed by the competitiveness of getting a good grade or having the best project. The seeming collaboration of teamwork in sports can be thwarted by the competition for getting a starting position or for receiving a college scholarship. I am not discounting the role of competition in our society; it will always exist at some level, and girls need to know how to live and thrive within it. But it is also important to recognize that cooperative collaboration has a genuine role to play in the emotional wellness of many girls, often as a complement to other areas of their lives in which direct competition is the rule.

Girls sometimes complain that their parents don't listen to them enough. These are likely, of course, some of the same teenagers who answer their parents' open-ended questions with single word responses ("Yes." "No." *"Fine."*). But this points out the importance of *creating* opportunities for collaboration and conversation. A recurring car ride or a weekend brunch or walk is simple to arrange but can create the opportunity and space to be profoundly communicative. When you least expect it (and likely when it is least convenient) is probably when that typically taciturn teenager starts talking with pointed enthusiasm.

EXERCISE

What are some ways in which you can create opportunities for collaboration with your daughter? It could be a mutually enjoyable activity like baking or cooking or gardening or could be taking a class together. Maybe you could work together to plan a local outing to an exhibit or a travel adventure. Perhaps you could make a date with other family friends to exercise together or do some sort of interactive community service. It could be a weekly brunch or teatime or monthly social or cultural activity. The first few times might be awkward, depending on your current relationship dynamic, but think of it as a work in progress.

CREATIVE COPING

When students come into my office for the first time, I ask them to name a creative hobby they enjoy. For many girls, it is an activity that they have long since put away or a craft that they don't get to do very regularly because of their busy schedules. When I work with girls, I encourage them to bring creativity back into their lives through whatever medium they choose. Some want to draw, write, paint, bake, sew, and practice photography. Others see playing cards or spending dedicated time with animal companions as their designated coping activities. Creative coping means different things to different people, and girls should be encouraged to explore and figure out what works best for them. One of the first girls I worked with had the goal of starting to sew again. She had a unique sense of style and a fashionista tendency that was about ten steps ahead of her peers. Her creations were both flattering and audacious, and at one of our subsequent meetings, she rocked a skirt of her own design.

Bringing creative opportunities into everyday life helps girls (indeed, it helps all of us) maintain integrity and individuality during stressful times. Creative coping gets our hands moving and refocused on activities that can have a meditative quality. It relaxes and invigorates us. The teenage years are so fraught with various ups and downs that actively establishing coping mechanisms that allow a healthy escape and use different skills can be the best way to handle stressful situations in a positive way. Even ten to thirty minutes a day, or time set aside once or twice a week, can make a noticeable difference. For some girls, taking a structured class may give them the initial motivation, whereas other girls prefer to keep it flexible so they can engage as they are able. Regardless, healthy creative coping opportunities are crucial aspects to developing and maintaining good emotional states for girls.

Examples of creative coping include:

- Painting, drawing, or other visual arts

- Knitting, sewing, or crafting

- Dancing

- Taking an art or photography class

- Making films or video editing

- Writing poetry or journaling

- Jewelry making

- Baking or cooking

- Creating music or practicing an instrument

NOTE: Creative coping is all about helping girls find something they love, not something they feel they are *supposed* to be doing. So if playing the violin feels like more of an obligation than an exercise, then it is not a creative coping mechanism for her.

EXERCISE

I call this the Playlist for Life exercise. I encourage teens to create two music playlists, one that's energizing and filled with music that makes them excited and bopping around, and one to help them to relax when they are stressed. Each list should have a minimum of ten to twelve songs that they truly enjoy listening to—the selection is up to them as long as it is music they prefer. The positive effects of music are well documented, and listening to favorite tunes can be a great coping mechanism for teenagers trying to sort out so many different things.[8]

COMMUNITY

Establishing a solid community in junior high and high school can seem daunting, especially because there can be different social minefields to navigate. But I encourage girls to think of their community with an expansive rather than enclosed view—one's community could include their family, friends who go to different schools, older role models and extended relatives, and even animal companions. Many children find enormous comfort in pets, and their role in emotional wellness should not be discounted. (One local psychologist looked at a mom after meeting with her daughter for a few sessions and said succinctly: "You should get her a dog.") Nonetheless, community can be made up of many different dimensions. As a part of building her own world, a girl needs to realize that she has the power to build her own sense of community that is unique to her and is a kaleidoscope of people that she interacts with in all the different facets of her life. And yes, in our digital world, some girls may find a community online that can be beneficial—though the opportunity for miscommunication and misunderstanding might be higher. I have seen girls completely expand their sense of community simply by more actively reflecting on ways that they could do so.

COURAGEOUS CONNECTIONS

Courageous connections refer to the notion of creating the opportunity for genuine and authentic relationships that foster growth and development. I use the word *courageous* because in our postfeminist, girl power world, it is sometimes wrongly seen as weakness to need help or appear vulnerable; needing help has been reduced to being needy. But, in fact, one of the strongest and most courageous things we can do is ask for help and to do so with a sense of confidence. It starts with understanding whom to reach out to.

Think about a girl who is struggling with her weight and has been told by her doctor that she is clinically obese. How can she find solutions without resorting to destructive reactive behaviors that might include drugs, stealth eating out of shame, or nutrient-deprived eating habits? What connections could she make to find a supportive environment and sound information about nutrition and health? Perhaps she doesn't think her parents know the proper information, or maybe she isn't comfortable sharing the details of her eating issues with them. She might be able to seek a nutritionist's or holistic health counselor's help or an outside source of health information, and then collaborate with her parents and let them know what she needs in terms of food options inside their home. Once she makes the connection and reaches out to find the person or place that can help her find healthy solutions, she can actively work to make the changes she wants in her life.

Creating a Core System of Support

Even if you assume your daughter knows she can turn to you for support, she may not always want to. Most of us, including girls, don't want to appear vulnerable in front of those we love the most (which is one of the reasons having a parent tutor a child is not always the ideal setup). Having a network can be crucial because there may be situations in which girls feel more comfortable talking to someone else (family doctor, therapist, clergy member, school counselor). It is important for this system to be in place *before* challenges arise. Parents and girls can answer the following questions separately to start the conversation, and these questions can be revisited as appropriate:

• Who is someone that you can trust and turn to when you have a problem that you need help with or are dealing with something that you have never dealt with before? Try to think of two or three different people or resources so if one isn't available, another could potentially be helpful.

• What are some positive behaviors that make you happy and calm you down? What are some things that you do when you are stressed that are probably not as good for you?

• When was the last time you were really stressed out? What made you so stressed?

• How did you handle it? What could you do differently that would be more positive?

• Where is a calming place for you to decompress and think through things and reflect? What makes that space so calming? Is there another place you enjoy as well?

• How would you go about seeking help for a problem that might be embarrassing or feel overwhelming? Where would you go? Who would you talk to?

‖‖‖‖‖‖‖‖‖‖‖‖‖‖‖‖‖

CHAPTER NINE

Physical Wellness

Our society sends girls mixed messages about what it means to be healthy. Does it mean looking good? Or feeling good? Or doing well in physical pursuits? It is all too easy, as part of the conventional, box-filling view of success, to think of a girl's academic performance and her college prospects as outranking every other dimension of her life. As long as those are on track, we are encouraged to think, it hardly matters what happens elsewhere. But if we are going to incorporate the insights of recent science as well as our and our girls' real-life experiences, we must take a much more holistic approach to cultivating girls' full development. A girl cannot be considered to be doing well if she has great grades, high standardized tests scores, and a long résumé of extra-curricular commitments but feels terrible about herself, is anxious all the time, and is continually exhausted or suffering from injuries.

My emphasis here is on three pillars of physical wellness: nutrition, exercise, and sleep. I am sure it comes as no surprise to hear that these three elements, individually and together, have a profound impact on girls' basic functioning. What we sometimes regard as typical tween or teenage girl behavior has a basis in neglected aspects of physical well-being. It's nearly impossible to be nice to others when you are feeling terrible inside. Any girl who has ever been irritable and lashed out at others for no apparent reason can recall how lots of little things can build up to create an overwhelming explosion. And any person who has ever dealt with a tired and cranky girl can attest to the bitter energy that is created by her bad moods. The eighth graders I met with universally laughed when recalling particularly morose and sullen moods and overwhelmingly agreed how horrible it felt to be awful to others. And yet, many of these girls (and the people around them) don't truly understand how much better they could feel by changing the way they approach nutrition, exercise, and sleep.

Nutrition

Many adult women admit to having had a long struggle with their relationship to food, and it may come as no surprise that girls younger and younger are dieting and developing the idea of restriction and avoidance when it comes to eating. Research shows that over 50 percent of high school girls and over 30 percent of elementary and middle school girls report being on a diet. Girls who diet have been shown to be twelve times more likely to binge than those who do not report dieting.[1] Similar to the way the notion of success in school is often reduced to standardized tests, scores, and grades, so the idea of good nutrition often narrows to counting calories, weight, and fat grams. Girls focus on what they can't or shouldn't eat and can get in a rut of eating the same self-regulated foods over and over. Recent CDC data reveal that nearly one in five girls admit that they have gone twenty-four hours without eating as a way of trying to lose weight or attempt to keep from gaining weight.[2] It's easy for girls to develop distorted relationships with food and cycle between extremes: stringent restriction and out-of-control binging. Nearly one in four high school–age girls are either overweight or obese, and it's not hard to see that this stop–start cycle of eating can wreak havoc on their bodies, minds, and spirits.[3]

As girls enter higher grades in school, it is not uncommon for them to be up late working on homework or socializing and then to get up early to prepare for school before their body has had time to properly rest. These girls try to camouflage their sleep-deprived state with caffeinated drinks and sugar-laden foods, which bring an unsustainable short-term energy jolt followed by a longer-term crash into exhaustion and anxiety. Perhaps they skip lunch because they don't feel like eating (or are socializing or studying). If they have athletic practice after school, they can be running on fumes before coming home and gorging on food before starting on their homework. At that point, they might be experiencing a mild food coma and need some sort of caffeinated or sugary jolt to get them through it. The cycle repeats itself.

Perhaps you think that your daughter is not one of those girls and that she eats fairly healthily. Or maybe you know that your daughter is going to the coffee shop every day and getting at least one latte, but you figure that there's very little you can do about it because she is already a teenager. Or perhaps the hot lunch options at school are the only available choice. Even some of the most progressive schools I visit serve lunches that center around processed food loaded with grease and preservatives. Many of the girls I've worked with don't immediately connect their lunchtime food choices with their bad moods or lack of energy later in the afternoon. Some girls who thought they were eating healthily were basing their choices on wrong or limited nutritional knowledge. If adolescence is the foundation for adulthood, many of these girls are starting out on shaky ground.

What I have found, though, is that girls *do* want to feel better and be more energized, especially as they deal with stressors from their academic and personal life that leave them feeling fragmented and out of place. Their bodies are undergoing rapid changes and are desperately in need of nutrients to promote the proper development of their body and brain. At the same time, girls often struggle to maintain an image of health—frequently by trying to lose weight in dangerous ways and developing a relationship of restriction and shame around what should be the pleasurable experience of eating and enjoying food. In the end, their bodies, including their brains, pay a high price.

CHANGING GIRLS' RELATIONSHIPS WITH FOOD

Our relationship with food begins at birth (or even in utero, based on the nutrients we absorb in the womb). And as we grow, our first food associations reflect our earliest models: parents, caretakers, and other familiar adults. As we in turn become role models, we need to examine the messages we send our girls and young women with our own food and eating choices.

As young children, many of us were encouraged to clean our plate instead of figuring out whether we were full. As a result, some of our initial messages about food were standards imposed on us externally. Women frequently admonish themselves for being good or bad based on their food choices. Girls are quick to observe and mimic their older siblings' or mothers' or friends' concerns about weight and body image. Some girls learn to see food solely as fuel and as something to be ingested standing up, in the car, or on the run. Others associate sugary or fatty food with happiness because they have grown up being treated to ice cream or donuts whenever they do something well or reach a certain achievement. Still others develop food-based fears and shame based on the constant barrage of conflicting messages sent by friends, peers, parents, and the media.

In an ideal world, girls and young women would see food as a source of both pleasure and sustenance. Several studies suggest that eating family meals can help promote health and wellness among students.[4] Encouraging girls to have healthy food relationships can start with having them take a more active role in meal preparation, to see and feel what fresh food is and where it comes from, and learn how different foods can be beautifully combined to support good health. More and more local farmers' markets provide an active food experience; making a weekly outing part of your regular experience can promote an expanding food-to-table awareness among young girls who might be obsessed with frozen yogurt and brightly colored energy drinks. Many of the girls I speak to bake treats for their friends or relatives from boxed mixes or premade cookie rolls. There is nothing necessarily wrong with this, but it's not the same experience as learning how to create something from scratch and experiment with different ingredients and options.

What are some ways to promote healthy food perspectives in the girls and young women in your life? It can be as simple as getting back to basics: to experience food in its elemental processes of growing, creating, and preparing. Tactile relationships with whole foods from a young age can potentially help girls develop more healthy food relationships. Some suggestions follow.

GARDENING

If you have a garden or space in your yard, create a project in which your daughter can have a little plot of land to create her own garden or grow a windowsill of herbs and other plants to be used in cooking. I've seen classrooms or homes with small garden plots in which the produce is rotated, depending on the season. If you live in an urban area, contributing to a community garden is also a good option. Gardening isn't only the act of planting and growing; all the little chores associated with it can be stress relieving, even weeding (!). Some of my most anxious students have admitted to finding solace in their garden plots and have experimented with planting different fruits and vegetables to see what transpires. There can be a special twinge of excitement from eating the cucumbers or tomatoes or spinach harvested from their own garden. Some food plants (such as kale or blueberries) are ornamental and can readily be given front yard status.

FARMERS' MARKET

If you live near a farmers' market, regular weekly outings can be used to encourage buying and preparing different varieties of fruits and vegetables. Getting to know the farmers encourages relationships with the entire food process and allows girls to expand their view of where food comes from and how they can incorporate a variety of whole foods into their daily eating. Pick an in-season fruit and/or vegetable every visit and try it in two or three different recipes. Depending where you live, some farms will also deliver boxes of fresh produce to your doorstep. Making a game out of finding a way to use everything in the produce delivery box can also add a little fun to the weekly routine.

WEEKLY OR MONTHLY MEAL PREPARATION

It's easy for any of us to get stuck in a rut when it comes to food. Creating a regular weekly or monthly time to try a new menu or recipe from scratch provides an opportunity for girls to experiment. Finding a way to track the experience (for example, in blog posts or on social media sites) and writing an accompanying story or paragraph can create a collaborative experience and provide humor for less-favorable outcomes and pictures and notes for good ones. The recipe doesn't have to be elaborate; try something individualized for your home and life. As Chef Gusteau says in the movie *Ratatouille*, "Anyone can cook!"

PRESENTATION

Give some thought to the eating environment in your home. Do you sit at the table to eat or is food eaten while doing several things at once? Is the television or computer on in the background? Is food on a plate or eaten straight from a box or bag? Talk to your daughter to find simple ways to create a peaceful or festive environment that works for all of you. Handmade place mats, fresh flowers, or candles and music can promote calm and change the energy and pace of the day.

EXERCISE

Reflect on your own food fears or rules. How did they develop? What are the foods that you currently eat most often? Have you rotated through different food ruts? When have you felt healthiest?

Now collaborate with your daughter to come up with ways to promote variety in eating and positive food relationships. Have her come up with a list of whole foods she would like to incorporate into new recipes, learn to create something from scratch, or plan a weekly farmers' market outing and let her choose in-season produce and find a new recipe to try. Or put a list of fruit and/or vegetables in a hat and pick out one to use as the "fruit/veggie of the week." Perhaps this can build on or incorporate the Game of Threes exercise from Chapter 4.

REFOCUSING ON BODY–MIND DEVELOPMENT

Unhealthy eating habits can sabotage girls' ambitions, whether they're studying for a big exam or trying out for varsity soccer. In one of the groups of girls I met with, every single girl had purchased the cafeteria's greasy oversize pizza even though most had high-intensity sports practice several hours later. When pressed, very few said that they regularly ate vegetables, because they didn't like them. Well-known physician and author Joel Fuhrman is concerned about the long-term well-being of adolescents, whose food choices provide the foundation for their health in decades to come. Indeed, Fuhrman argues that the diseases that show up decades later have their roots in our diet choices as adolescents. Fuhrman believes there are three particularly important components for the healthy physical and mental development of teenage girls: consuming healthful omega-3 fatty acids, maintaining proper vitamin D levels, and eating phytochemicals in micronutrient-dense foods.[5]

Healthful omega-3 fatty acids have repeatedly been shown to be crucial for healthy brain development and function. Omega-3s are found in nuts and seeds like walnuts, chia seeds, ground flaxseeds, and pumpkin seeds. Although omega-3s are also found in many different kinds of fish, concerns surrounding mercury levels in seafood can make fish a less desirable choice. Many girls avoid nuts because of the high fat content (though some of these same girls regularly eat pizza, nachos, and sugared drinks) or simply because they haven't been introduced to the idea of incorporating them into their diet. Omega-3 supplementation can be as simple as adding ground flaxseed to oatmeal in the morning, making chia seed muffins, or eating walnuts or pumpkin seeds as a midmorning snack. It's all about making simple switches that expand the range of good choices.

Vitamin D is known as the sunshine vitamin, because a certain level of exposure to direct sunlight is needed for proper absorption. Vitamin D has many important health effects. It is needed for proper calcium absorption, which is important for long-term bone development and to reduce the risks of osteoporosis. Vitamin D deficiencies also lead to muscle weakness and may increase the risk of certain kinds of cancer.[6] More recent studies also suggest a potential link between low levels of vitamin D in adolescents and increased rates of mental health issues such as depression and anxiety.[7] So many girls and young women are struggling with emotional anxiety and depression that making sure vitamin D levels are sufficient can be one important part of an overall wellness plan.

Phytochemicals from micronutrient-dense foods are also crucial to healthy growth and development. Micronutrients are all the vitamins, trace minerals, phytochemicals, and food factors that living organisms need in small quantities for proper functioning but do not produce themselves. Phytochemicals are the chemicals in plants that are responsible for, among other things, the vibrant colors of vegetables. In his book *Eat to Live*, Fuhrman talks extensively about the importance of using micronutrient-rich foods such as green and colorful vegetables, fruits, and legumes as a basis for a healthy diet.[8]

By consuming more micronutrient-rich foods, girls are able to restore their energy and health. A girl's skin, hair, and eyes all feel and function differently based on the constant absorption of subtle nutrients to nourish her on a daily basis. What girl doesn't want shiny hair and smooth skin? Nutrients definitely play a role. In an ideal world, the more vitamins and minerals we can obtain directly from foods, rather than from supplements or artificial means, the better.

Most parents complain that their girls (and boys) don't like to eat vegetables. But many people don't like vegetables because they have never really tasted fresh vegetables. Again, getting access to fresh organic produce can make a big difference. Even though availability can vary depending on where you live, there are almost always opportunities, one way or another, to find good fresh food. Repeated exposure is key; most kids need to try a food many times before being able to decide whether they like it. In other countries (most of western Europe comes immediately to mind), kids eat vegetables far more readily because they become accustomed to them as a normal part of their diet. There are so many different ways to eat vegetables, and a little kitchen fun can also go a long way. For instance, kale chips are one of my favorite healthy treats; they're delicious and easy to make at home.

EXERCISE

You and your daughter can both keep a food/mood journal for a week. Write down everything you eat and also write down your mood. Use whatever adjectives (or emoticons) you feel appropriate, and see if you can each find a connection between your food choices and how you feel. Maybe you forgot to eat and ended up being cranky or you had a sugar- and fat-laden meal of processed fast foods that left you in pain a few hours later.

Then look up a list of omega-3- and micronutrient-dense foods. Each month, have your daughter come up with one or two foods to incorporate into your diets at the expense of other foods that aren't serving her as well. Try them several different ways in different recipes—for instance, if broccoli is the food of the month, it could be sautéed, added to a baked dish, or served raw with dip.

HEALTHY FATS FOR A HEALTHY MIND AND BODY

One recurring theme I hear from many girls who are concerned about their physical appearance is that they avoid all fats. They view fat as the mortal enemy, and fail to realize that some fats are necessary for proper growth and development. They eat packages upon packages of fat-free snacks as a way of avoiding fat at all costs. But this trade-off typically results in increased consumption of sugars and highly processed carbohydrates, which can actually be more responsible for gaining weight than fat is. Eating easily digested carbohydrates tends to spike insulin, which in turn, when blood sugar levels drop, reignites appetite. Often, the serving size of a typical fat-free food is minuscule, and it's easy to keep eating far beyond the recommended portion.

More important, though, young girls and adolescents are at a key age where healthy fats play a crucial role in their brain and body development and potentially their emotional and physical wellness. Research shows that there is a marked difference between good fats needed for healthy growth and development and bad fats that contribute to many of the diet-related health challenges down the road. Monounsaturated fats include avocados, nuts, and seeds as well as olive, canola, and peanut oils and are recommended as a part of a solid overall diet. Polyunsaturated fats, which include the omega-3 fatty acids noted above, are found in vegetable oils, flaxseed, and walnuts and are recommended because they help lower both blood cholesterol levels and triglyceride levels.[9] Saturated fat and trans-fatty acids found in animal products and processed foods are to be limited or avoided.

SHORT-TERM FIXES VERSUS LONG-TERM SUSTAINABILITY

Most adolescent girls can recall a time when their energy levels crashed and burned, and I have yet to meet any girls who joyfully reflect on that experience. More and more, girls reach for caffeine and sugar-laden drinks to help get them through a day filled with energy highs and lows. Among my students, I see junior high students who drink double or triple lattes to help them get focused for morning tests or have coffee before afternoon diving practice as a way to become energized.

But, as legal addictive stimulants, coffee and other caffeinated drinks quickly put us into overdrive when we are really running on empty. Many girls use caffeine as a short-term fix when they are energy depleted even though it contributes to poor sleep quality later on.

Looking for long-term sustainability in eating patterns is a good goal for anyone. As they begin to emerge, the good effects—consistent energy levels replacing physical and emotional highs and lows—provide motivation to continue improving. Some suggestions follow.

BUNDLING BREAKFAST

Some girls get up so late or are busy getting ready for school for so long that they don't think that they have time for breakfast or their stomachs might not yet be ready to consume anything. Encourage them to try some warm water and lemon juice (ideally, freshly squeezed lemon juice from half a lemon) to neutralize their stomach before eating anything. Then they can bring something to school to eat during their first or second class (if the teacher allows it) or during the morning break.

Healthful smoothies can be an appealing way to broaden girls' dietary horizons and can even be made the night before to save time in the mornings. There are lots of recipes available that include fruits, vegetables, nuts, and other nutrient-dense foods, and for girls who are still averse to eating certain kinds of foods, being creative with the recipe can be part of the fun.

Girls who are constantly running too late to have breakfast can help think of three or four simple alternatives to keep on hand, packed ready to go. Soy yogurt, a flaxseed muffin, or apples and almond butter are all good options that can promote variety across the daily diet. Ideally, even a quick breakfast will include some protein and complex carbohydrates for sustained energy at the start of the day.

DECAFFEINATING AND HYDRATING

In my office, hot tea quickly became popular among the students after I created a fun tea basket filled with different herbal tea brands and flavors. Like vegetables, many girls who think they don't like herbal tea haven't really been exposed to what's available. Drinking a hot cup of tea can be a calming coping way to take a break and transition away from a rough day. Sometimes, making it attractive is all in the presentation.

Teeccino, which is readily available in health food stores and larger grocery stores, provides a caffeine-free alternative to coffee that retains the roasting flavor and aroma and is a great trade-off. For girls and young women who are trying to make the transition away from over-caffeinated drinks, I suggest gradually swapping Teeccino for coffee (and yes, it does the trick!).

Sometimes exhaustion actually masks dehydration; think about a plant that hasn't been watered and wilts. We also seem to wilt when we are not properly hydrated. A good option is coconut water, which has the natural electrolytes important for rehydration. Regular water is great too, and getting a reusable water bottle that is attractive and lively can promote its actual usage (and be ecologically friendly).

PACKABLE LUNCH OPTIONS

Hot lunch or cafeteria-purchased lunches can be easy and popular options for those who are running out the door or short on time. (Though, lunch can always be made the night before.) Look at the options provided by your daughter's school and at what she is actually eating. Most lunchtime bestsellers are sugar- and fat-laden choices that can lead to midafternoon emotional and energy crashes.

Focus on encouraging gradual changes to promote long-term patterns of sustainable energy. Asking a girl to go instantaneously from five days a week of hot lunch to bagged lunch from home might be a tough sell. One option is to divide the week into home-meal days and school-lunch days: Two or three days a week lunch is brought from home. Have her come up with a few choices she would eat readily and try a few quick meals at home. Having a selection of lunches that can be easily assembled the night before is important for this to be workable. Perhaps a weekend baking project can provide the dessert for a week of lunches.

HEALTHY SNACKING

When I ask my students what they eat when they get home from school, many can't even remember. Some are so ravenous (because they didn't eat lunch) that they eat everything and anything in sight. Many complain that the more healthful choices in their kitchen aren't things they actually like. As Manhattan-based nutritionist Jodi Greebel notes, teenagers tend to go after crunchy snacks—so tortilla chips and salsa or guacamole, crudités or pita chips with hummus, almond butter on crunchy apples, or celery sticks with raisins and a nut butter can be sustaining choices to help them make the transition into homework time.[10]

EXERCISE

Spend one afternoon cleaning out your cupboards with your daughter. Set the timer for two hours and throw out everything that has expired or is not a good choice. Then sit down together and come up with a list of foods your daughter would eat for breakfast, lunch, and snacks that would help her sustain her energy levels throughout the day. Pick a few to make sure you always have something both nutritious and appealing on hand.

ACNE AND NUTRITION

Most girls struggle with acne in some form at some point over their teenage years and often rush to see doctors and dermatologists for quick-acting pharmaceutical solutions. Or they become convinced that drug-store remedies, some which can be loaded with irritating chemicals that can end up being counterproductive, will provide relief. But few girls think of diet as an important element in developing or preventing acne. New evidence suggests that what we eat can indeed influence how clear our skin is or isn't.

Recent studies, for example, have pointed to a link between dairy consumption by teenage girls and increased levels of acne.[11] There is also some evidence that if a person has a gluten allergy, the inflammation that results from the intolerance can aggravate preexisting acne. And high glycemic index (GI) foods (ones that cause insulin levels to spike) can also increase levels of hormones that exacerbate the skin's oil production.[12]

If any of these kinds of foods seem to bother a girl's skin, it is quite easy to find alternatives without losing nutritional value. Calcium, for example, can be derived from green leafy vegetables. Hemp milk, almond milk, rice milk, and soy milk are all healthful and tasty options to cow's milk. Gluten-free breads and snacks are now commonly available. And eating fewer simple or highly processed carbohydrates is a good idea for most people, not just for those suffering from acne.

VITAMIN F (FOR FUN)

Food choices, nutrition, and health are loaded topics for many girls and young women. I truly believe that a nutrient that is essential for overall health but is overlooked on the charts of calories, protein grams, fat intake, and RDAs of vitamins and minerals, is *fun*. We need to enjoy our food to bring sustenance and vitality to our lives. How we choose to spend our lives moment to moment represents how we want to build our lives. Encouraging girls to figure out what they find fun and making it an essential part of their daily lives is as important to overall health as is eating more leafy green vegetables.

Fun should be considered an emotional nutrient, and if we regard its daily allowance as essential as we do those of trace vitamins and minerals, then we will go a long way to promoting the overall health and wellness of our girls.

So, in addition to thinking about food and nutrition, encourage your girls to spend some time figuring out how to bring more fun into all of your lives. Maybe it's through spontaneous adventures or planned activities, or perhaps you'll find a way to make mealtime more fun with funny questions or silly surprises. Loosen up, embrace creativity, and allow your girls to do the same.

Exercise

In Sanskrit, the term *Ahimsa* refers to the principle of being nonviolent and having thoughtful consideration for all living things. In yoga, the term encompasses the importance of compassionate kindness to everyone and everything. As girls and young women, we know how easy it is to be tough on ourselves; we do not give ourselves the same compassion and understanding that we give to others, especially when it comes to our physical wellness.

If we think about it in the context of Ahimsa, then, true exercise should be something that helps us gain flexibility, endurance, and strength and improves our overall health and wellness without causing us pain and injury. But this does not describe the experience of most girls in most sports, which is often marked by a *no pain, no gain* philosophy. Girls are told they need to exercise to be healthy, but many of the extreme forms of exercise and athletic participation now deemed normal quickly cross the line from being helpful to harmful.

THE RISE OF SPORTS

In the last few decades, girls' participation in organized sports and athletics has reached record numbers. Indeed, girls and young women benefit in many tangible ways from their participation in sports and athletics. In addition to promoting teamwork, athletic participation gives many girls an outlet to release stress, maintain healthy weight and body mass, and increase cardiovascular and muscular strength.[13] Many girls learn important lessons about communication, collaboration, and friendship on the playing fields much more effectively than in the classroom. Recent studies have suggested that there are lifelong health benefits from high school sports participation. Sports participants even tend to complete more years of post–high school education. Many women look at their time as part of a team as among the happiest experiences in their young lives.

At the same time, it has been only in the last several decades that girls' athletics have taken on their current high level of competitiveness and become a maze filled with politics, injuries, and the constant stress of never feeling good enough. In many instances, girls ask their bodies to do things that they are not designed to do, leading to physical and emotional distress as well as overuse and other types of injuries. It's not just in soccer or organized high school sports, but it's in the high-intensity aerobics, obsessive weight lifting, and conditioning that push an extreme ethic of more, better, and bigger. While the tangible benefits are many, there has also been a painful rise in the number of sports-related injuries and surgeries. We don't know what all the long-term effects and damage of the overtraining and injuries can be, and we need to step back and reflect on how we evaluate sports in relation to the lives of girls and young women. Looking beyond merely athletic involvement to understand the entire scope of health-building exercises is important for promoting lifelong physical wellness.

SINGULAR FOCUS AND SPECIALIZATION

When Hailey first walked into my office her freshman year of high school, she had a razor-sharp dedication to playing soccer. She played on a traveling club team, and spent more than twenty hours a week in training, either at soccer practices on the field or in conditioning training with a personal trainer. Her weekends were spent traveling to tournaments; between her club team and her high school team, she spent nearly forty-eight weeks a year focused on soccer. Her summers were spent at camps doing intense conditioning, and simple adventures like taking the day to head to the beach had to be planned around practices and soccer-related commitments. She had little need or desire to pursue any other interests because her goal of playing at the Division I level absorbed her attention and was all she wanted. Beyond soccer and school, her free time for any other pursuits was limited; her singular focus was impressively serious but also enormously limiting. In her junior year, I asked her what she liked to do for fun besides soccer, and she looked at me as though I had three heads. Even my suggestion to find another activity for a mere hour a week was met with an icy stare.

Like many girls, Hailey's goal of excelling in soccer made her feel that she needed to specialize early on. But such narrow focus always comes with risks of overuse and burnout. By the time she tore her anterior cruciate ligament (ACL) late in her junior year and was forced to have surgery, she had spent most of her high school career fixated on playing soccer. With soccer, her future seemed set. Without it, she was lost.

After the initial shock of her surgery and rehabilitation, Hailey regrouped a bit and made some tough decisions. She decided to give up playing soccer right before her senior year. With her newfound time, she started to dabble in other interests, joining the school newspaper, going to the beach with her friends, and learning how to relax. Slowly, a more colorful character began to emerge from her once stoic demeanor. She lightened up, and with a twinge of regret, she told me that, though she wouldn't have changed her experience on the soccer field, she now realized she had sacrificed a typical high school experience to her single-minded commitment. Now she was glad that she was able to spend her senior year just being a teenager.

Excelling at anything generally requires a considerable amount of hard work and effort, which in itself is a good thing. But the fact that many girls and young women are now *required* to specialize in their athletic participation is disconcerting for several reasons. These girls are still growing and developing but in many cases are being forced to specialize far earlier than ever before. Physically, by focusing on one or two sports so soon, they reuse the same muscles and become more prone to injuries and long-term damage. More than that, though, this specialization sends the same psychological message of asking girls to be finished projects. Instead of being able to experiment and try new things and grow and explore, they are forced to commit to something before they are able to expand their options, and in doing so, the sport that they once found to be fun and stress-relieving can become serious, stressful, and overwhelming.

> More than that, though, this specialization sends the same psychological message of asking girls to be finished projects.

OVERDOING IT WITH TWO SPORTS AT ONCE

Many high-level student athletes are juggling the expectations and workouts of playing multiple sports at once, leaving them even more prone to injury and exhaustion. Some girls participate in sports whose season hasn't ended before the preseason of their next sport begins, and even though they aren't supposed to be doing multiple workouts, their concern for losing favor with coaches or losing their spot on the team leads them to overcommit. Or girls are playing a club sport outside of school (for example, volleyball) while also participating in a school team (say, field hockey). On some evenings, these girls will have school practice from three to five thirty, eat dinner in the car, and practice the second sport from six to eight. When they finally get home, they are physically and mentally exhausted. Thanks to the double workouts, these girls may be teenagers spending more hours training than would be legal for them to work in some states. Parents often become complicit in these overscheduling arrangements because they don't want to deny their girls the opportunity to work out and succeed in an area they love. In some cases, the allure of potential college scholarships can also cloud objective judgment. But what often happens is that these girls end up putting themselves through more work than their bodies can handle, all while trying to balance the demands of school and other obligations.

GIRLS' INJURIES

We now put extreme expectations on girls (and boys) to play longer, harder, and more decisively at earlier and earlier ages. Recent studies show that girls are five times more likely than boys to sustain concussions, and girls tend to experience concussion symptoms for longer than their male counterparts. Girls are also four to ten times more likely to have ACL knee injuries. A recent much-cited study from Ohio State University concludes, "In high school sports played by both sexes, *girls sustained a higher rate of concussions, and concussions represented a greater proportion of total injuries than in boys.*"[14] In my office, we see several students a year who are sidelined from both school and sports as a result of surgery and subsequent rehabilitation. Much of the athletic training involves having girls train in ways that are not meant for their body structure. Michael Sokolove's 2008 *New York Times Magazine* piece titled "The Uneven Playing Field" looks at the increased number of girls struggling with torn ACLs.[15] As he notes, the physical differences between girls and boys that start to appear during puberty are thought to be a factor, perhaps related to girls' wider hips and different knee angles.

Though research continues to try to pinpoint why exactly girls suffer more injuries than do boys, we also are just starting to look at the lifetime effects of these injuries and patterns of extreme overexertion.

Other research notes that the recovery process from concussions is different for girls, who may require more time than do boys.[16] Scientists are just beginning to look at the long-term impact of concussions and are trying to explain why female soccer players suffer from more concussions than do male soccer players. And although some exercises can help girls learn how to properly build up their muscles to prevent some injury, ACL injury rates still remain high among girls and young women.[17] For girls' athletic participation to be truly beneficial, these problematic and potentially chronic effects need to be addressed and remedied.

NUTRITION AND EXERCISE

For many girls and young women, exercise and athletic participation can quickly cross over from being beneficial to being harmful, especially when proper nutrition is overlooked. When this happens, sports can get caught up in, and be part of what generates, long-term life imbalances. Some girls can become confused and overwhelmed at the way that their body changes in response to both their athletic training and puberty. Some female athletes will restrict their food intake as their musculature changes in response to their new workouts. I've seen high school soccer players whose muscular thighs no longer fit into their old jeans become horrified and cut their calories to lose weight.

ATHLETICS AND EXERCISE AS ANOTHER ACHIEVEMENT
Just as it becomes easy to fall into the box-filling trap of achievement with academic and extracurricular pursuits, it can be all too easy to fall into the routine of pleasing others when it comes to exercise and athletics. The heightened level of early competition can also alienate girls who

want a less intense experience. Think about the student who is trying to balance the expectations of multiple coaches or is dealing with the increased competition of trying to make the starting roster on the school team or gain the coveted spot on the prestigious traveling club team. The benefits of cardiovascular exercise and collaborative team-work disappear as goals behind the more intensely encouraged ambition to succeed in more visible ways. What once was fun and stress relieving now becomes another element of perfectionistic achievement.

PROMOTING MORE MOVEMENT THAN JUST EXERCISE

All girls can and should enjoy the wellness benefits of living a lifestyle that, quite simply, promotes movement. Regardless of whether they prefer team sports or singular pursuits or if they want something that is regulated and routine or spontaneous and sporadic, realigning the spirit of exercise with a lifestyle that promotes increased movement is one that can set girls up for lifelong health and wellness. In the book *The First 20 Minutes*, author Gretchen Reynolds asserts, "Humans are born to stroll."[18] Indeed, much of her book talks about how less is more and that simply moving more on a regular basis can make a long-term impact on overall health.

Walking or riding bikes instead of driving and taking the stairs instead of the elevator are actions that seem simple enough but are often overlooked in our frenetic and fast-paced world. We have long been aware of the overwhelming health benefits of walking more, but so many of us think we are in such a hurry that we can't afford to take the time to walk to get where we're going. I always find it peculiar how many people (I have been guilty of this myself) drive to the gym and get on a machine when just getting to the gym on foot could be quite a workout. It has become ingrained that we need to visualize our exercise as another task or appointment to be scheduled and to be performed in a specialized exercise setting, but in fact one of the most widely healthful habits we can adopt is that of regarding everything we *do*—all of our daily actions—as a series of opportunities to move in ways that our bodies need. The change in perspective, from time-slotted exercise to holistic movement, is probably the single most effective decision we can make for physical fitness. To promote more movement with girls, an inviting way is to make it a game. There are different ways of keeping an eye on fitness—from a simple pedometer to a computerized tracker like Fitbit, which tracks movement, sleep, and exercise—some of which can potentially make it fun. Fitbits and similar devices can also track distance traveled and calories burned and thus work well for athletes who need to make sure they are eating enough with ramped up workouts (though, again, it can cross over from fun activity to obsession, so be mindful of what works well for your daughter).

GET OUTDOORS

Emily came to my office from her freshman to senior year in high school. Her mother had died when she was young, and she lived with her stepmother, father, and two younger half siblings. It was easy to see that Emily's relaxed and easygoing nature did not mix well with her more assertive, hard-charging stepmother. At school, Emily blended into the background of any classroom so much that many of her peers didn't even realize she was in their science or English classes. She was a student who rarely spoke up, and her few attempts to join high school sports teams were met with lukewarm results. She wanted to be more active but felt that the opportunities were limited and that she didn't fit into the niche prescribed by her athletically oriented high school.

Given Emily's precarious relationship with her stepmother and her own indifferent school and athletic experience, I suggested she try an outdoor hiking adventure as a summer excursion before her junior year in high school. Her stepmother thought it would be a great way to get Emily more self-motivated to pursue excellence and signed her up almost immediately. I thought it would be a great way to get some fresh air and be inspired by the natural beauty of the outdoors and also to meet some new kids in a different environment from the school setting.

Even I was shocked at the transformation that occurred after

Emily's outdoor adventure. She realized that she actually enjoyed hiking and spending time outdoors, which she had never really done before. She came back with a sense of optimism and enthusiasm that spread into every aspect of her life. She became more confident and reflective and found ways to become more involved and organized at school.

Spending more time outdoors is a simple way to change a day, a mood, or a way of thinking. Girls obviously don't need a specific outdoor wilderness camp or adventure to increase their time spent outdoors, but it might be the right opportunity for some girls to try something new. Even in parts of the country where the weather makes it difficult to spend time outdoors for a good part of the year, taking advantage of every possible opportunity can make a difference. Because so much of schooling and socializing now occurs indoors, it's important to find ways to build outdoor movement into girls' lives; walking instead of driving and going for a bike ride instead of the gym can promote the breathing, thinking, and reflecting and open up a new perspective.

YOGA

A yoga teacher who works with elementary and middle school students diagnosed with attention deficit hyperactivity disorder (ADHD) recently commented on how many of the students look forward to shavasana, which is also known as "corpse pose" and is the final resting pose that closes most yoga practices. These kids love the stillness of this final peaceful resting position. Even at their young age they are fully aware that the constant movement and busyness of their days can create stress that feels overwhelming.

In my work, I see many girls who play a sport or are active in some way but very few who have ever tried yoga beyond a few yoga sequences as part of an athletic warmup. It is rare to meet a girl who has done yoga on a regular basis. Yoga poses and concerted sequences can provide stress relief, and the physical and physiological openings can promote a sense of calm and concentration. Given the emotional anxiety and related struggles that many middle and high school girls experience in the course of their daily school experience, yoga can provide a good antidote to help them clear their minds and refocus. Conscious breathing and mindfulness, two key elements in any yoga practice, can offer perspective to the academic and social challenges a girl may feel she faces off the mat.

Yoga has incredible emotional and physical benefits, and studies are just starting to look at the impact that a regular yoga practice can have on adolescents in relation to weight loss, mental health, and mood disorders. There are many different styles of yoga, so girls can truly find something that works for them based on their age and needs, and more and more children's yoga classes are becoming available nationwide. Initial findings are promising, and it can be a consistent and inexpensive way to bring calm to an otherwise overscheduled and bustling life.[19]

THE FUN NUTRIENT IN EXERCISE

When it comes to being active and getting exercise, it should ideally be enjoyable; have girls come up with a few ways that they can make their workouts more fun. Maybe it's new colorful laces in their sneakers or a more comfortable pair of headphones. Little things can make a big difference. I recently bought some electric blue sneakers that are so bursting with color that it's hard not to smile every time I put them on. A friend, who for years loathed any form of exercise, fell in love with Zumba classes and now plans her schedule around them. She would take the classes even if they weren't exercise, which is pretty ideal. Encourage girls to find a partner (perhaps a parent) and create a fun challenge involving taking the stairs instead of the elevator or walking or biking instead of driving. Inspiring more overall movement as a lifestyle and coming up with ways to make it more fun can build a foundation for long-term wellness rather than short-term starts and stops.

EXERCISE

What are different ways to promote more natural movement in daily or weekly life? What is a simple swap you and your daughter can make to increase your physical activity? List three different ways to incorporate more movement into your lives, and find three ways to make movement more fun. Running stairs at a local outdoor space? Put together upbeat music playlists? Come up with simple solutions together.

IIIIIIIIIIIIIIIIIIIIIIIIIIIIIIIIIIIIIIIIIIIIIIIIIIIIIIIIIIIIIIIIIIIIIIIIIIIIIIIIIIII

Sleep

As I've mentioned, being sleep deprived challenges our ability to learn, our memory, our emotional state, our immune system, our ability to cope with stress, as well as our metabolism. And yet, more and more girls who feel stress about their schoolwork, their weight, and whether they will remember all the state capitals are not getting enough sleep. Because they are sleep deprived, their skin looks tired, their eyes look tired, and in general they function less effectively. Quite simply, they are denying themselves the opportunity to look good, feel good, and work well.

So many girls complain that they have trouble falling asleep at night and their early wake-up times cut into their sleep cycles just as they were getting comfortable. It is true that the teenage years are associated with a later sleep–wake cycle in general. In terms of improving sleep quantity and quality, I've found it particularly effective to give students access to information and allow them to educate themselves. When they see the results of the most recent research on sleep and its effect on learning and emotional processing, they often become far more receptive to finding solutions to help their own lives be better. Getting more sleep takes some active effort, especially in a world in which we are constantly connected electronically and otherwise. A few suggestions follow.

AFTERNOON SNACKS/EVENING SLEEP CONNECTION

As adults, we generally recognize that having caffeinated drinks after a certain hour can directly affect how and when we sleep. Some girls who get up early for school and then experience an afternoon crash before homework or sports practice don't realize that the caffeine or sugar jolt that they reach for after school can be detrimental when they are trying to wind down at the end of the day. Girls who are having trouble falling asleep should look first at what they are eating when and then at what they can swap for potentially better options.

SCHEDULING TO MAKE SLEEP A PRIORITY

Each spring, high school students plan their classes for the following year. There is often an unspoken (or spoken) pressure to sign up for the most challenging class load possible to appear competitive to colleges. But most high school counselors note that taking five AP classes or honors classes leaves students, mathematically, very little time to sleep if they are also involved in extracurricular activities and have a social life. I often see this double-edged sword in conversations with parents. Many are worried about their child's sleep habits and academic pressures, and yet, when it comes down to it, they yield to the pressure. Out of fear of insufficient achievement, they encourage their kids to sign up for a combination of classes and extracurricular activities that will be overwhelming and emotionally detrimental for their overall wellness.

Just as it's okay to say no to a dinner party or weekend excursion when you are exhausted, girls need to learn that it is okay to say no to an overwhelming number of obligations. Parents need to encourage their children to create an individualized schedule that will allow them to get rest, pursue personal interests, and be challenged. If the high school counselor said that each AP class averages seven hours of homework a week, that is twenty-eight plus hours per week if your daughter takes four AP classes. Realistic? Healthy? What's right for her? Remember: What's overwhelming for one person is par for the course for another, so individualized approaches are key.

TECHNOLOGY CURFEW

Just as putting technological gadgets away can be helpful for girls when they are trying to concentrate on doing their work, it can also be essential when it comes to getting a sound night of sleep. Many high school girls readily admit that they will go to bed with their phones nearby, and wake up in the middle of the night or stay up far past their desired bedtime chatting or texting with friends. Some girls admit that they would want their parents to enforce this curfew because even with their best intentions, they are not always able to regulate themselves. Enforcing a technology curfew, by which phones and other technological devices are kept out of the bedroom after a certain hour, can help.

BEDTIME ROUTINES

Bedtime rituals typically get lost along the way from early childhood to adolescence. But reinstating a more mature version of these nightly traditions can be a useful way to make the transition from activity to rest. Turning off all screens (TV, phone, computer) even thirty minutes before bedtime can make a big difference, and consciously spending some time coming up with a set routine that promotes calm *and* allows the next morning to go more smoothly is ideal. Here are some ideas for bedtime routines:

Putting cell phones and other gadgets in the charger or technology box

Preparing everything necessary for a good breakfast

Making snacks and lunch for the next day

Packing up backpacks and putting them by the door or in the car

Setting out an outfit for the next day

Taking a shower or bath so the following morning's primping and prepping are minimized

Listening to relaxing music

Writing in a journal or reading for pleasure

Sipping a cup of calming herbal tea

If your daughter is having trouble falling asleep, have a collaborative conversation about ways to make the hour or so leading up to bedtime a time to unwind so that she can fall asleep more readily.

WHITE NOISE MACHINE

For some girls, the sheer frenzy of the day makes it tough for them to fall asleep in total silence. Or they are so sensitive to the sounds around them that every dripping faucet keeps them awake. A white noise machine might work wonders in giving them enough audible distraction to achieve better sleep and relaxation. For others, smooth classical jazz or other instrumental music might relax them into a sounder slumber.

WEEKENDS AS SLEEP-IN TIME

There is so much information telling us that sleeping in on weekends is a bad thing because it disrupts our sleep rhythms and that we should ideally get up at the same time each day. But most teenage girls would agree that they don't like getting up early five days a week, so allowing them to sleep in as they please on weekends can be crucial for reclaiming some of their built-up sleep debt. If there isn't a reason for them to get up early (and be really careful about what is a good reason to get up early on weekends; it should be something *they* want to do, not something *you* think they should want to do), letting them sleep might be a way for them to regain a few hours from their sleep deficit.

THE FUN NUTRIENT IN SLEEP

Just like nutrition and exercise, there should be a fun element in how girls get to sleep. A girl's bed and bedroom should be a restful sanctuary, and sleep should be something she looks forward to. What are ways it can be more fun? Are there soothing colors in her bedroom or is it a blank space? Is there a fun bedtime ritual you can reincorporate from when she was younger or can you work to start a new one? What does her bedscape look like? What does she go to sleep with? Pillows, stuffed animals? Do family pets sleep in her bed, and if so, how does that affect her sleep? Has her bedroom been updated for her current age and needs? Does she have comfortable pajamas that she loves to sleep in?

EXERCISE

Have your daughter track her sleep quality for a week (again, a computerized tracker like a Fitbit might make this more fun). She should track when she went to bed, approximately how long it took her to get to sleep, and how she felt she slept. Was her sleep adequate? Did she feel like she got too much or too little? If it was too little, what prevented her from getting more? Come up with some solutions together.

||||||||||||||||||||||

CHAPTER TEN

Spiritual Wellness
Reflecting and Connecting

In her book *Things I Want My Daughters to Know*, lifestyle philosopher Alexandra Stoddard writes, "Going inward is our way to see the light, to experience greater clarity and harmony."[1] In the previous chapters, we've looked at the many ways that girls' reactivity to the external expectations can mire their ability to develop their own inner voice and personal sense of authenticity. One of the most damaging potential losses is the way so many girls prevent themselves from cultivating their own sense of spirit and promoting their own spiritual wellness.

Spiritual wellness can be easily overlooked in the achievement arms race. For some, spirituality refers to religious beliefs and values, and for others, it does not. Regardless, a girl's spiritual wellness is inherent for her healthy growth and development. I refer to spirituality in the most inclusive sense, as a way that encompasses the core values that a person chooses to live life by. It incorporates appreciation for what we can learn, and how we can broaden our perspectives and ideas rather than simply stay where we are comfortable. For girls who struggle with so many external messages, focusing on their own spiritual wellness can guide them in their decision making and give them a sense of comfort when dealing with challenges and opportunities.

Like self-care and emotional wellness, the importance of spiritual wellness is sometimes overlooked until there is some sort of crisis. Teenage girls trying to figure out their own identity can easily become weighed down on focusing on the here, now, and self. Spiritual wellness enables girls to expand their perspective and worldview, cultivate self-knowledge, and encourage positive personal transformation. It can help girls find an inner strength and resilience in time of challenge and change, which is crucial given all the external and internal upheaval girls face going through adolescence. Promoting spiritual wellness and personal understanding is a way for girls to create and frame their point of view on their life and values.

Editing, Reevaluating, and Letting Go

Girls' interests change and evolve as they are exposed to new opportunities, possibilities, and discoveries. What may have been their favorite thing ever in junior high may be little more than a passing interest by the time they reach high school. Girls can become overwhelmed when they keep adding without subtracting, whether the adding has to do with activities, obligations, or physical belongings. Much of the overscheduling that girls experience is a result of adding more activities and obligations without taking the time to let other obligations fall by the wayside; it's all about too many yeses and not enough nos. It's easy to become literally and figuratively cluttered and confused when we

> It's easy to become literally and figuratively cluttered and confused when we hold on to things past our own personal expiration date.

hold on to things past our own personal expiration date. For girls, learning how to subtract with grace and become flexible to evolve can be one of the most challenging aspects of cultivating a sense of authentic personal spirit.

Editing personal space can be particularly powerful. Changing colors, reevaluating the objects and photos on display, and deciding what we include in our personal space can affect us emotionally and spiritually. Editing and reevaluating doesn't have to be expensive or overwhelming, and girls can creatively come up with ways to decorate on a less-is-more budget. Finding inexpensive frames and putting fancy paper, meaningful sayings, or photo collages in them can be a simple and fun way to decorate wall space.

For some girls, letting go and moving on can seem overwhelming and slightly terrifying, because they don't have enough life perspective to realize that editing and reevaluating can be some of the most powerful ways to promote spiritual growth and wellness. Parental and adult support can be helpful, and making a yearly or otherwise regular tradition of reevaluating can serve a meaningful purpose as they undergo personal transformations. Girls, like all of us, have a personal threshold as to how much they can hold and can quickly overflow with obligations if they take on too much without editing with integrity. When girls allow themselves to edit their lives, they give themselves permission to let go of what is no longer useful for them and make physical, literal, and spiritual space for things that are useful. It could be as simple as cleaning out childhood soccer league trophies, dropping an activity or class that is no longer of interest, cleaning out the clothes closet, editing childhood collections, or making proactive decisions about how and with whom girls spend their time. To welcome in new opportunities and evolve as individuals, girls need to give themselves permission to let go of the past and appreciate it for what it was and is.

EXERCISE

Ask your daughter to reflect on the places in her life that could use editing: her physical space (room, clothes, or general stuff), her schedule (extracurricular activities, social obligations), and her relationships (friendships, acquaintances, romantic relationships). Encourage her to visualize what she would like to say no to in order to be able to say yes to something new.

Then, if appropriate, set aside a few hours over the summer or a school break to do some physical editing: what to donate, what no longer serves a purpose, and what needs to be replaced.

||||||||||||||||||||||||||||||||||||||||||||||||||||||||||||||||||||||||||||||||||||||||||||||||

Hearing, Understanding, and Appreciating the Inner Voice

When girls are focused on attaining some sort of perfection, they can quickly fall into the trap of taking and placing blame on others and themselves when things don't work out the way they want. It becomes easy to take a blaming approach instead of being gracefully held accountable and taking ownership of one's own options, opportunities, and possibilities.

Common blaming refrains include the following:

That teacher hates me and that's why I am not doing well in the class.

It's all her fault that our project went horribly.

I am so bad at math and never do well on tests.

The coach is so unfair in not giving me more playing time (not making me a starter).

My mom is so mean!

Blaming is energy misspent for all involved. When girls blame others or themselves, they misappropriate their (often limited) personal resources and avoid looking inward to figure out how they can move forward from a situation that may be less than ideal. In doing so, girls can realize the personal benefit of acting with grace even when they are tempted to react otherwise. Seeing situations for what they are and evaluating what they can do and how they can proactively respond in a way that remains true to their own personal values and integrity can help girls feel empowered in times that might be otherwise wrought with uncertainty, pain, or annoyance.

There's something to be said about gut instincts and that sinking feeling a girl gets when she is at a party and she senses all is not good; she needs to know that instinct should be listened to. With so many outside influences telling her how to think and act in so many different ways, a girl needs to develop and trust her inner voice.

In reading this, you may be thinking that is all well and good, and it would be great if I could convince my teenage daughter to accept responsibility gracefully and figure out proactive solutions, but sometimes when she is yelling/crying/sulking/blaming it is not really possible to do anything but try to defuse the situation without too much long-term damage. But again, it's all about timing. Helping girls realize that they do have options in all situations about how they react and choose to engage or disengage ultimately allows them to reinvest their energy in ways that allow them to develop their intuitive perspective.

For example, when a girl comes into my office blaming someone else or herself, I ask her to step back and answer these questions:

- Who are you blaming and what is the subject of your blame?

- How could you more proactively address the situation? (I ask her to list the options and consider which one is best.) What is your gut instinct?

- How can you take responsibility or ownership gracefully? (I remind her that it is not a matter of blame or fault but rather a chance to behave in a way that allows her to move forward.) From this new perspective, what are some ways you could have reacted and what are some things you can do now?

• What should you do next?

These questions don't need to be asked word for word, especially if it would do little more than garner an eye roll, but it can be a useful way to start a conversation looking at past events as well as future challenges. Will teenage girls always act with grace? Not likely. It is all about progress, not perfection.

Reflection of the Outward and the Inward Messages

It's natural for us to get our sense of values from external sources when we are younger, but as we grow up, we may find that some of those values might hold true for us, while others might not. In today's always-on socially connected world, it can seem impossible for girls to step back and create their own philosophy and values for living irrespective of the many outward messages they receive. Many adults are still asking these tough questions, so it's doubly challenging for a preteen or teenage girl to do so. But it is possible, and because so many girls are facing difficult issues earlier than did previous generations, this values-based and inward reflection seems more essential than ever before.

Rosalie's parents, Marnie and Robert, both had demanding, high-paying careers. The creature comforts of their monetary success included private school education for all three of their children, exotic vacations, and beautifully appointed luxuries. It was typical for one of them to be traveling or working late, though they both made remarkable efforts to have one parent home at all times. Marnie and Robert valued the financial stability their careers gave them, even though both readily admitted that they didn't find their work fulfilling or satisfying. Both had few if any hobbies or interests outside of their work, and dinner conversations centered on office politics, potential projects, and new opportunities. In high school, Rosalie's perfectionist habits caused her to struggle with anxiety, depression, and disordered eating habits. By the time she sought outside support, Rosalie was in the midst of a crisis and felt conflicted between the values her parents held important and her own developing sense of spirit.

Over the next few years, Rosalie started to cultivate her own personal values and made the inward journey of figuring out her own sense of understanding, given the world she lived in. She began to explore her own sense of what she valued and how she felt about her own personal truth. Rosalie realized that although she felt grateful for the many opportunities her parents' financial success and stability afforded her and her siblings, she longed for a life's work and purpose that brought her inward joy as well as outward comforts. And even though that seemed idealistic to her parents, she wanted to challenge herself in her efforts to align her goals with her sense of purpose and personal values when it came to potential work and career possibilities. During college, she took internships and opportunities that she thought might be fulfilling and purposeful to her, and ended up working in a position in arts education. She learned to live with less financial comfort and wean herself from her parents' support, because she wanted to live her life without the attachments of a life she couldn't afford to provide for herself. It took her a few years, but she managed to do it.

Ultimately, a girl's spiritual wellness is grounded in her understanding of her own personal integrity. In their attempt to build their own worlds, girls need to understand that their beliefs are theirs alone and don't need to necessarily be approved by anyone. It can be scary for girls to sort though their own values and can be uncomfortable if they are not necessarily in line with those around them, but it ultimately can be a grounding and empowering process.

EXERCISE

This is a simple exercise your daughter can do on her own or with you.

Have her look over the list of twenty-seven commonly held values listed below and select the five or ten values she considers most important. Feel free to add other ones, if you like. Then, have her look at the list and reflect on how those values are practiced in her own life and how she might want to incorporate them even further. For example, if one of her values is gratitude, she might ask herself how she practices gratitude in her daily life toward herself and others. What more could she do to live by this value?

Honesty	Open-mindedness
Integrity	Spontaneity
Compassion	Flexibility
Perseverance	Faith
Thoughtfulness	Simplicity
Gratitude	Authenticity
Family	Humility
Community	Humor
Empathy	Optimism
Generosity	Realism
Kindness	Creativity
Wisdom	Courage
Love	Complexity
Tenacity	

CULTIVATING THE CONNECTION

When Rachel was younger, her family spent Sundays going on a morning hike in nature followed by a family breakfast filled with spirited conversation and meaningful reflection. Her parents didn't have any particular religious affiliation, as each parent was culturally raised in households of different faiths and neither parent felt much connection to his or her religious upbringing. Rachel's parents saw their Sunday morning tradition as a way for them to promote their own spiritual wellness. As Rachel grew older, she joined a local youth group at the neighborhood synagogue as a way to explore her own faith and develop her own connection to her spirit and spirituality. The community of the youth group, coupled with the activities and opportunities, gave her the chance to reflect and explore her own set of values in a way that nothing else did. She looked forward to the Wednesday evening gatherings and various weekend outings and came away from her youth group experience with a heightened sense of self and new perspective to consider. In the summers, she became involved with a youth group–affiliated service group and summer camp. Though her parents were initially surprised by her dedication to the youth group and its related religious activities, they realized that Rachel's own spiritual development might be very different from their own.

We all deserve to have a place or experience that helps to ground us; for some, it may be attending weekly religious services, whereas for others listening to music, baking or cooking for themselves or others, performing selfless service, being in nature, or staring at the ocean might be most effective. What works for one person may not work for someone else, which is why cultivating spiritual wellness is such a personal endeavor. One girl who lived near the water would leave her family's Sunday morning church services and go down to the ocean to stare at the water and listen to the waves crashing. Sometimes she would listen to her favorite music, and other times she would just allow the sound of the waves to be her main musical distraction. The key to cultivating a sense of connection is that girls are able to leave and disconnect from the everyday space of the mundane and be permitted to freely discover new perspectives, ideas, and views. There may be several places that allow for that space for transformative meditation, reflection, and renewal. For a high school student I worked with, baking quietly in her kitchen in the dark of night gives her that sense of transformative calm.

Remember, what works for one person might not work for another, and what works at one time might not necessarily work at another.

EXERCISE

Ask your daughter to list two to five places or experiences that she has found calming or grounding. It may require some reflection, and perhaps she has yet to find a place, but this exercise can get her to start thinking about what brings her a sense of tranquility and peace.

The Overlooked Beauty of Selfless Service

Paige was a high school junior who was truly at odds with her high school experience. She couldn't stop counting the days until graduation, and her outward physical beauty belied her inner shyness and insecurity. She had never really recovered from a sophomore year betrayal by friends who ostracized her and left her to spend lunchtime sitting at the periphery of a table at which she didn't feel she truly belonged. Though she had a good deal of perceived popularity in part because of her family's wealth and her own petite, blond, perky good looks, she really could not wait to leave the superficiality and cattiness that pervaded her high school experience. It didn't take long after we started working together for me to realize what a wonderfully thoughtful person Paige was, and I wanted to help her find a sense of fulfillment outside of her high school experience. At that point, she didn't participate in any activities and was pretty disengaged with the entire school process. When I asked her to list some things that she enjoyed and felt that she was good at, she mentioned working with younger kids. I suggested she look into an after-school program that provided tutoring and care to elementary school students in a neighboring community. I helped her apply, and she signed up to volunteer one day a week.

A few months later, I was surprised to learn from the center's director that Paige was coming in two to three days a week; the children loved her, and though she was somewhat quiet and reserved with the adult staff members, she consistently went above and beyond to meet the children's needs. Even though the center was a twenty- to thirty-minute commute, she was one of the center's most reliable and responsible teen volunteers. When I asked her about her experience at the center, she quietly exclaimed that she enjoyed it, and I could see a bit of a smile creep back into her face as she shared a few stories. When she was filling out her college applications, I had to remind her that she could include her volunteer work at the center as an activity, and she continued volunteering well into the fall and spring of her senior year. For Paige, her selfless service at the after-school center was a good antidote for the stress she felt from her high school experience.

In Chapter 4, I talked about selfless service as a way of helping girls develop their own sense of purpose. For girls like Paige, selfless service can help them get beyond the everyday fragmentation of adolescence. Selfless service doesn't just help promote purposefulness; it also encourages spiritual wellness.

Disconnection from the Everyday

One of the most central tenets of feng shui is that there must be a balance of yin energy (stillness) with yang energy (action). For overscheduled and overcommitted girls, spiritual wellness may require an active disconnection or deactivation from outward influences, especially when they are going through a particularly trying time. Thoughtful reflection generally requires full concentration and cannot be readily interrupted by blurps and beeps. It may be as simple as going for a walk without technological interruptions or leaving the phone and other gadgets away when on a weekend vacation or weeklong excursion. It could be a silent meditation in the morning, or a weekly silent family dinner (likely, the first time you have a silent family dinner is the first time a normally morose teenager has something they are dying to share).

EXERCISE

How could a technology mini-vacation (or even daily escape) be incorporated into your family's life? It could start small, as a daily time without email or social networking and a corresponding escape into an experience that is personally fulfilling (for example, an art project, a gardening activity, a walk by the water, a hike, a writing project, or an act of selfless service). Figure out where and how that could happen, and what would make the experience meaningful.

THE IMPORTANCE OF FUN IN SPIRITUAL WELLNESS

There is a certain simple joy in acts of spontaneity—running into a friend and catching up, or deciding to visit a museum and take a walk around the park on a day that was earmarked for other plans. Of course, there is certain comfort and calm that comes with being organized and making plans; indeed, I work with students on organization and time management, but there is an equal happiness that comes from impulsively doing something just for fun, with no rhyme or reason other than the day is beautiful and the picnic blanket needs a grassy green field to sit on.

Each of us has a different definition of what I like to call frivolous fun. In the middle of working on this book one morning, I needed a break and left my home office and walked down to the skating rink near my apartment in San Francisco, picking up a hot chocolate along the way. I hadn't really skated for years, and I have no idea why I was so immediately enthused at the idea of getting on the rink again except that some of my favorite childhood memories are at the skating rink. The mini-adventure was pure fun (after I regained my sense of balance). I was able to clear my head and put a simple smile on my face, which carried me through the day and into the next with a sense of kid giddiness. It was as if I had done something mischievous by taking a break, when in actuality I just allowed myself to have a little fun. It's easy for spontaneity to fall by the wayside when girls are overscheduled and overorganized; the point of learning organization and time-management strategies is to give them the option to have *more* unplanned fun.

There is a certain spiritual component to allowing ourselves to be flexible and play and have fun for no reason other than it is what we feel like doing. It can bring calm and comfort in trying times and bring the opportunity to cope and expand perspective and possibilities. Skating around the ice rink allowed me to relax and ultimately made my writing and work more focused. Frivolous fun is all about girls recognizing that they can't and shouldn't be on all the time, that they need the opportunity to say yes to something that speaks to them in the here and now.

EXERCISE

Have your daughter brainstorm a list of things that she would consider to be fun. It could be going to an art museum, visiting the park, taking a drive to a neighboring downtown, or exploring a new venue. This varies, of course, by where a girl lives and what her resources are, but play and fun can be achieved in many different ways. Have your girl write her choices on individual slips of paper and put them in a hat, jar, or other container. Then, once or twice a month, designate a spontaneous fun afternoon (it could be a surprise determined at the last minute) and have her reach into the jar and pull out the day's activity (of course, if it's raining, you may not be able to go to the park . . . or maybe you could?).

DIVINE INSPIRATION

Each girl has her own personal style. Filling her world with words, scenes, ideas, and pieces that she loves can make her conscious of her choices, abilities, and opportunities. The recent popularity among teenage girls of social media sites like Pinterest and Tumblr speaks to the fact that girls (and women!) want the opportunity to express their beliefs, dreams, and sense of style. In a world in which they are constantly being influenced by outside sources, they still long to individuate themselves.

When we surround ourselves with things we like, it heightens our senses. Encouraging a girl to create an intentional personal space can build a sense of calm and appreciation. Perhaps it is the top of a dresser, or maybe a corner in which she can place her favorite beanbag chair and comfortable blanket to curl up in. She can choose what colors, objects, photos, and words feel right to her based on her own intuitive sense, and she can focus on what is beautiful to her. Maybe her space includes plants, flowers, or pictures of friends. Perhaps she has her favorite colors or meaningful sayings on display.

Each girl uses her personal space—whether she has her own room, shares a room with siblings, or has very limited or nonexistent space—as an extension of identity formation and a source of personal inspiration. Having her actively think through what she would include in such a space forces her to evaluate and reevaluate what she wants to bring into her world and can help her look at life with more proactive optimism rather than a reactive pessimism. Though some girls already do this naturally, encouraging them to instinctively recognize what is meaningful and moving to them is another way they can develop their sense of spirit.

EXERCISE

Encourage your daughter to set aside a small space as her own to curate however she pleases. Before starting, encourage her to brainstorm about what she would want the space to include and what objects, sayings, photos, or colors would fit her desired image. For a girl who may not have her own space, perhaps she can create the space virtually or as a storyboard.

|||||||||||||||||||||||

CHAPTER ELEVEN

Conclusion

Implementing the Strategies

After going through all the tips and strategies in this book (and learning more about teenage girls than you ever thought imaginable), you might be a little overwhelmed! You know your home and family dynamics best, so you're probably thinking about which strategies could be easily implemented in your situation (like creating a study space) and others that might take time and effort (getting your daughter to minimize technological distractions, perhaps). As with anything else, making sweeping long-term changes takes time, especially when we are talking about a preteen or teenage girl who is trying to juggle the demands of school, friends, and family. There will inevitably be starts and stops, but try to focus on helping to create an environment that promotes a sense of purpose, fun, and wellness. Allow opportunities for your daughter to regularly stop, regroup, refresh, relax, and refocus.

I hope that as you read the previous chapters, you were able to think about how you could work collaboratively with your daughter to incorporate some of the strategies in your home and life. I wrote this book as a primer to help parents work with their daughters and create individualized solutions. Again, two important caveats: you know your daughter best, and you likely know what strategies would be most helpful and what might be the best way to introduce some of these strategies. Change takes time, and the more gradual and consistent you are about promoting changes, the more likely they will become a part of your lives rather than be a short-lived experiment.

Remember the Importance of Attitude

Sometimes girls can be tough to understand, and they can be even tougher to figure out! Resist the urge to become frustrated, and focus instead on collaborating, communicating, and finding solutions. It could be as simple as stepping back and allowing your girl to envision her life and then encouraging her to become a proactive builder of her own big, enriching, invigorating life. Getting angry or annoyed is just wasted energy; instead, figure out ways to concentrate your efforts on helping your daughter brainstorm ways to make her life both simpler and more enriching, all at once.

It's Okay to Outsource

You may have read the previous chapters and thought there was no way that your daughter would ever respond well if you tried to introduce some of the strategies to her. You know your family dynamics best, and perhaps an aunt, older cousin, or family friend or mentor would be a better fit to promote certain conversations. Indeed, that is one of the (many) reasons students find their way to my office. But, you might be pleasantly surprised! The exercises in the book can be easily done in tandem, and many are casual conversation starters. Many girls tell me they wish someone had asked them the questions and done exercises in this book, so, there may be hope!

Any Day Is a Good Day to Start

Although it might be easier to implement some of these strategies at the beginning of the school year or in January when change is in the air (!), I truly believe that any day is a good day to start. After all, this book is all about discovering purpose and promoting wellness, and any day is a good day to begin the road to finding more joy and happiness.

Sample Six-Step Strategy

The six-step plan I present here is merely a suggestion; I encourage you to come up with an individualized solution based on your daughter's needs and the time of year. There are exercises throughout this book for you to pick and choose from, and this six-step strategy incorporates many, but not all, of them. You may choose to personalize the strategy with alternative exercises or do the exercises in a different order altogether. For instance, some of the academic study skills might be moved to later if she starts the steps when school is out of session. Your daughter might adapt some strategies right away, and others might take time. In general, two weeks is a good amount of time for each step, but again, there is no set formula; each student is different. Even though you move on to Step Two or Three, for instance, revisiting the exercises in Step One may be important. I hope you and your daughter can use these steps as part of an overall journey toward active communication and overall health and wellness. I hope the process will encourage changes as you all go through the exercises. Above all, be patient, optimistic, and open to the good things to come.

STEP ONE

- Time Management Sheet and Weekly Flow Chart (Chapter 4)

- Discuss academic and personal purposes and goals (Chapter 4)

- Buy necessary supplies (Chapter 5)

- Organize physical and digital binders and use a written planner (Chapter 5)

- Create a study space and Technology Box (Chapter 5)

- Fun activity: collage with personal values and purpose

STEP TWO

- Game of Threes exercise (Chapter 4)

- Implement two-hour homework blocks (Chapter 5)

- Create a system in which homework is done on the night it's assigned (Chapter 5)

- Physical wellness exercise: track food, sleep, and mood (Chapter 9)

- Fun activity: playlist for life

STEP THREE

- Start working toward Game of Threes exercise (Chapter 4)

- Active learning exercise (Chapter 4)

- Look at selfless service opportunities (Chapter 4)

- Look at the master calendar and reduce unfulfilling activities (if applicable) (Chapter 4)

- Incorporate strategies for studying for quizzes and tests (Chapter 6)

- Social wellness activity: television and technology digest—what is your daughter watching? (Chapter 7)

- Fun activity: cooking with new ingredients

STEP FOUR

- Incorporate active reading and active studying strategies (Chapter 6)

- Entrepreneurial exercise (Chapter 4)

- Physical wellness: clean out the cupboards; create breakfast, lunch, and snack opportunities (Chapter 9)

- Emotional wellness: read and do exercises for the C's of Success (Chapter 8)

- Social wellness: friendship values exercise (Chapter 7)

- Spiritual wellness: create a personalized space (Chapter 10)

- Fun activity: creative coping

STEP FIVE

- Focus on a particular strategy that needs extra attention

- Revisit academic and personal purposes and goals; revise if necessary

- Physical wellness: create an optimal sleep environment (Chapter 8)

- Emotional wellness: create a system of support (Chapter 8)

- Spiritual wellness: values exercise (Chapter 10)

- Fun activity: schedule time to do something fun to reduce stress (hike, yoga class, cook, bake, craft)

STEP SIX

- Revamp study space based on needs (Chapter 5)

- Take a technology or texting break

- Physical wellness: promote breakfast (Chapter 9)

- Emotional wellness: community web exercise (Chapter 8)

- Social wellness: sexting and bullying exercise (Chapter 7)

- Spiritual wellness: journal and reflection (Chapter 10)

- Fun activity: visit the farmers' market or create a windowsill herb garden

ACKNOWLEDGMENTS

First and foremost, I would like to thank all the students with whom I have been so fortunate and privileged to work throughout the years. And to their parents, thank you for the opportunity to work with your children—I truly consider it a gift.

Many thanks to my phenomenal early readers and friends who supported this book (and this writer!) through various stages. Judy Rothenberg, thank you for your supportive comments that always provided thoughtful perspective and sparked new insights. Jeanmarie Cahill, I am forever grateful for your wit, wisdom, and genuine encouragement. Margaret Miller, thank you for all your support and caring on this and every other project in my life. Alice Kleeman, thank you for your friendship and for your generous feedback on many chapters of this book. Laura Zimmerman, thanks for your support in the midst of everything else—much appreciated. Sarah Cheyette, thanks so much for your warmth and graciousness, as well as your valuable feedback on an early draft of this book. Your insight as both a mother and a pediatric neurologist was invaluable. Sarah Goldberger, thanks so much for your positive enthusiasm and optimism, as well as your brilliant marketing strategies. Kaitlyn Nagi, thank you for being the eleventh-hour research assistant extraordinaire—I am so grateful for your efforts. Annie, thanks for working me through some chapters that were especially challenging, and offering advice and encouragement as needed.

There were many people who gave so generously of their time to be interviewed for this book. I hold each of our conversations in such high esteem and am truly thankful: Matt Walker, Mary Carskadon, Meighan Wilson, Jane McClure, Deborah Gee, and many parents and students who preferred for their contributions to be anonymous—you know who you are, and thank you. Susan Marquess, thank you for your continued support. Brenda Dyckman, thank you for all your help with my earliest Girls Groups, and for all your support throughout the years. Emily Dickson, thank you for being the most amazing office manager and all-around fabulous person. I appreciate all you do to make everything run smoothly, and everything is just more fun with you around. Ellen Truxaw, your genuine kindness and warmth are unparalleled—I wish you much success in all your future endeavors.

To Priscilla Gilman, thank you kindly for your early assistance with the proposal. And to Richard Prud'homme, thank you for your insights on the early draft of this book.

To the wonderful people at Perigee, John Duff and Marian Lizzi, who were supportive of this book from the very beginning and whose editorial insights were invaluable. I am so appreciative of your efforts in every stage of this book's journey—from inception to completion (and title-searching somewhere in between!). Thank you to Candace Levy for her wonderful copyediting, and to Lauren Becker for all her help with final details.

To my fabulous agent, Julie Just at Janklow and Nesbit, your genuine enthusiasm, remarkable support, and extra efforts are unparalleled. I feel so lucky to get to work with you. Thank you for everything.

And finally, this book is a result of my own sense of personal purpose, and I want to thank my parents, Amir and Bahereh, for teaching me the importance of character, perseverance, and unwavering integrity. I am forever grateful for your efforts. To my sister, Allia, thanks for always offering a humorous perspective on the girl world and for keeping it real.

NOTES

||||||||||||||||||||||||

INTRODUCTION

1. Sam Roberts, "For Young Earners in Big City, a Gap in Women's Favor," *New York Times*, August 3, 2007, www.nytimes.com/2007/08/03/nyregion/03women.html.

2. Jennifer D. Britz, "To All the Girls I've Rejected," *New York Times*, March 23, 2006, www.nytimes.com/2006/03/23/opinion/23britz.html.

3. Roberts, "For Young Earners in Big City, a Gap in Women's Favor."

4. Institute for Women's Policy Research, *Hot Topics: New Study: Men Earn More Than Women within Nearly All the Most Common Occupations*, Institute for Women's Policy Research, April 17, 2012, www.iwpr.org/press-room/press-releases/new-study-men -earn-more-than-women-within-nearly-all-the-most-common-occupations.

5. *A.D.A.M. Medical Encyclopedia*, s.v. "Adolescent depression," www.ncbi.nlm.nih.gov/ pubmedhealth/PMH0002486.

6. David Knopf, M. J. Park, and Tina P. Mulye, "The Mental Health of Adolescents: A National Profile, 2008," National Adolescent Health Information Center, University of California at San Francisco, 2008, http://nahic.ucsf.edu/wp-content/uploads/ 2008/02/2008-Mental-Health-Brief.pdf.

7. Ibid.

8. National Adolescent Health Information Center, "Fact Sheet on Suicide: Adolescents & Young Adults," University of California at San Francisco, 2006, http://nahic.ucsf.edu/ downloads/Suicide.pdf.

9. Rachel Simmons, *The Curse of the Good Girl: Raising Authentic Girls with Courage and Confidence* (New York: Penguin, 2009).

10. S. M. Suldo, M. M. McMahan, A. M. Chappel, and T. Loker, "Relationships between Perceived School Climate and Adolescent Mental Health across Genders," *School Mental Health* 4, no. 2 (2012): 69–80.

1. THE PERFECT GIRL MYTH

1. Jenny Anderson and Peter Applebome, "Exam Cheating on Long Island Hardly a Secret," *New York Times*, December 1, 2011, www.nytimes.com/2011/12/02/education/on-long-island-sat-cheating-was-hardly-a-secret.html.

2. Daniel E. Slotnik and Richard Pérez-Peña, "College Says It Exaggerated SAT Figures for Ratings," *New York Times*, January 31, 2012, www.nytimes.com/2012/01/31/education/claremont-mckenna-college-says-it-exaggerated-sat-figures.html.

3. Stephen P. Hinshaw with Rachel Kranz, *The Triple Bind: Saving Our Teenage Girls from Today's Pressures* (New York: Ballantine, 2009), pg. 112.

4. Judy Rotherberg, in-person interview on November 15, 2011.

5. Tanya Caldwell, "A First Draft of 2012 Admissions Decisions at Dozens of Universities," *The Choice Blog, New York Times*, April 16, 2012, http://thechoice.blogs.nytimes.com/2012/04/16/college-admits-2012.

6. Jack Hough, "College: Big Investment or Big Risk?," *Wall Street Journal* May 5, 2012, p. B5.

7. Diana Zuckerman, "Little Girls Become Women: Early Onset of Puberty in Girls," *The Ribbon* 6, no. 1 (2001).

8. Ibid.

9. Peggy Orenstein, *Cinderella Ate My Daughter* (New York: HarperCollins, 2011), p. 91.

10. "Candie's Debuts Spring Marketing Campaign Starring Actress, Lea Michele," *PR Newswire*, January 25, 2012, www.prnewswire.com/news-releases/candies-debuts-spring-marketing-campaign-starring-actress-lea-michele-138036358.html.

11. *Introducing Lea Michele for Candie's*, YouTube, January 25, 2012, www.youtube.com/watch?v=Xpv_pYKY8aA.

12. Diane E. Levin and Jean Kilbourne, *So Sexy So Soon: The New Sexualized Childhood, and What Parents Can Do to Protect Their Kids* (New York: Ballantine, 2008), p. 69.

13. Jane Gross, "In Quest for the Perfect Look, More Girls Choose the Scalpel," *New York Times*, November 29, 1998, www.nytimes.com/1998/11/29/nyregion/in-quest-for-the-perfect-look-more-girls-choose-the-scalpel.html?pagewanted=all&src=pm.

14. American Psychological Association, "Report of the APA Task Force on the Sexualization of Girls," 2008, www.apa.org/pi/women/programs/girls/report.aspx.

15. Victoria J. Rideout, Ulla G. Foehr, and Donald F. Roberts, "Generation M^2: Media in the Lives of 8- to 18-Year-Olds," Henry J. Kaiser Family Foundation, January 2010, www.kff.org/entmedia/upload/8010.pdf.

16. "U.S. Teen Mobile Report: Calling Yesterday, Texting Today, Using Apps Tomorrow," *Nielsonwire*, October 14, 2010, http://blog.nielsen.com/nielsenwire/online_mobile/u-s-teen-mobile-report-calling-yesterday-texting-today-using-apps-tomorrow.

17. Rideout et al., "Generation M^2."

18. Dan Strober, "Multitasking May Harm the Social and Emotional Development of Tweenage Girls, but Face-to-Face Talks Could Save the Day, Say Stanford Research-

ers," January 25, 2012, http://news.stanford.edu/news/2012/january/tweenage-girls
-multitasking-012512.html. Roy Pea and Clifford Nass, "Media Use, Face-to-Face
Communication, Media Multitasking, and Social Well-Being Among 8- to 12-Year-Old
Girls," *Developmental Psychology* 48, no. 2 (2012): 327–36.

19. Rideout, "Generation M²."

20. Ibid.

21. "About Formspring," www.formspring.me/about.

22. Centers for Disease Control and Prevention, "Skin Cancer: Indoor Tanning," November 2, 2011, www.cdc.gov/cancer/skin/basic_info/indoor_tanning.htm.

23. National Sleep Foundation, "2006 Sleep in America Poll: Summary of Findings," 2006, www.sleepfoundation.org/sites/default/files/2006_summary_of_findings.pdf.

24. Centers for Disease Control and Prevention, Division of Adolescent and School Health, "Youth Risk Behavior Surveillance System: Selected 2011 National Health Risk Behaviors and Health Outcomes by Sex," 2011, www.cdc.gov/healthyyouth/yrbs/pdf/us_disparitysex_yrbs.pdf.

25. National Sleep Foundation, "How Much Sleep Do We Really Need?," www.sleepfoundation.org/article/how-sleep-works/how-much-sleep-do-we-really-need.

26. Eileen Patten and Kim Parker, "A Gender Reversal on Career Aspirations: Young Women Now Top Young Men in Valuing a High-Paying Career," Pew Social and Demographic Trends, April 12, 2012, www.pewsocialtrends.org/2012/04/19/a-gender-reversal-on-career-aspirations/?src=prc-headline.

27. John Medina, *Brain Rules: 12 Principles for Surviving and Thriving at Work, Home, and School* (Seattle: Pear, 2008).

28. Larissa Faw, "Why Millennial Women Are Burning Out at Work by 30," *Forbes*, November 11, 2011, www.forbes.com/sites/larissafaw/2011/11/11/why-millennial-women-are-burning-out-at-work-by-30.

2. SO MANY WAYS TO BE BOXED IN

1. Alexandra Robbins, *The Geeks Shall Inherit the Earth* (New York: Hyperion, 2011), p. 42.

2. As research shows, girls' brains tend to mature one to three years faster than boys' brains, which can make a big difference in junior high and high school.

3. PARENTAL ATTITUDES AND APPROACH

1. Stanford Report, "'You've Got to Find What You Love,' Jobs Says," June 14, 2005, http://news.stanford.edu/news/2005/june15/jobs-061505.html.

2. Patti Neighmond, "Working to Stop Teens Texting behind the Wheel," Pew Internet, May 10, 2010, www.pewinternet.org/Media-Mentions/2010/Working-To-Stop-Teens-Texting-Behind-The-Wheel.aspx.

3. This is the finding of Carol Dweck, whose research on success has shown that it's the perspective on success—whether you believe it's innate or developed—that actually determines the level of success. See her *Mindset: The New Psychology of Success* (New York: Random House, 2006).

4. Anne Kadet, "Job Hunting: When Parents Run the Show," *Smart Money*, February 27, 2012, www.smartmoney.com/plan/careers/job-hunting-when-parents-run-the-show -1328630501076/?link=SM_clmst_sum.

4. BREAKING DOWN THE BOXES

1. William Damon, *The Path to Purpose: Helping Our Children Find Their Calling in Life* (New York: Free Press, 2008), p. xiii.

2. Ibid., pp. 41, 43.

7. SOCIAL WELLNESS

1. C. Brené Brown, *The Gifts of Imperfection: Let Go of Who You Think You're Supposed to Be and Embrace Who You Are* (Center City, MN: Hazelden, 2010), p. 94.

2. Louann Brizendine, *The Female Brain* (New York: Morgan Road, 2006), p. 31.

3. Henry J. Kaiser Family Foundation, "Daily Media Use Among Children and Teens Up Dramatically from Five Years Ago," News Release, January 20, 2010, www.kff.org/ entmedia/entmedia012010nr.cfm.

4. Amanda Lenhart, Mary Madden, Aaron Smith, et al., "Teens, Kindness and Cruelty on Social Network Sites," Pew Research Center's Internet & American Life Project, November 9, 2011, http://pewinternet.org/Reports/2011/Teens-and-social-media .aspx.

5. Christine Haughney, "Seventeen Magazine Vows to Show Girls 'As They Really Are,'" *New York Times*, July 3, 2012, http://mediadecoder.blogs.nytimes.com/2012/07/03/ after-petition-drive-seventeen-magazine-commits-to-show-girls-as-they-really-are.

6. Candace Smith, "Teens Post 'Am I Pretty or Ugly?' Videos on YouTube," *ABC News*, February 23, 2012, http://abcnews.go.com/US/teens-post-insecurities-youtube-pretty -ugly-videos/story?id=15777830.

7. Somini Sengupta, "'Big Brother'? No, It's Parents," *New York Times*, June 25, 2012, www.nytimes.com/2012/06/26/technology/software-helps-parents-monitor-their -children-online.html?_r=2&smid=tw-share.

8. J. R. Temple, J. A. Paul, P. Van Den Berg, et al., "Teen Sexting and Its Association with Sexual Behaviors," *Pediatrics and Adolescent Medicine* (2012), http://archpedi.jamanet work.com/article.aspx?articleid=1212181.

9. Ibid.

10. "Hannon's 'Sexting' Legislation Signed into Law," NewsLI.com, September 27, 2011, www.newsli.com/2011/09/27/hannons-sexting-legislation-signed-into-law.

11. Centers for Disease Control and Prevention, "Youth Risk Behavior Surveillance System: Selected 2011 National Health Risk Behaviors and Health Outcomes by Sex," 2011, www.cdc.gov/healthyyouth/yrbs/pdf/us_disparitysex_yrbs.pdf.

12. L. Owens, R. Shute, and P. Slee, "'Guess What I Just Heard!': Indirect Aggression among Teenage Girls in Australia," *Aggressive Behavior* 26 (2000): 67–83.

13. L. Owens, R. Shute, and P. Slee, "'It Hurts a Hell of a Lot . . .': The Effects of Indirect Aggression on Teenage Girls," *School Psychology International* 21 (2000): 359–367.

14. Amy Chua, *Battle Hymn of the Tiger Mother* (New York: Penguin Press, 2011).

15. Elisa Benson, "35 of Our Best Flirting Tips," *Seventeen*, July 2012, www.seventeen.com/love/advice/best-flirting-tips.

8. EMOTIONAL WELLNESS

1. *Karen Owen's Duke List Powerpoint*, YouTube, October 8, 2010, www.youtube.com/watch?v=hahYUHkw9KY.

2. Andrew Luo, "Duke Admits 3,105 to the Class of 2016," *The Chronicle*. March 30, 2012, www.dukechronicle.com/article/duke-admits-3105-class-2016.

3. Centers for Disease Control and Prevention, "Youth Risk Behavior Surveillance System: Selected 2011 National Health Risk Behaviors and Health Outcomes by Sex," 2011, www.cdc.gov/healthyyouth/yrbs/pdf/us_disparitysex_yrbs.pdf.

4. David Knopf, M. J. Park, and Tina P. Mulye, "The Mental Health of Adolescents: A National Profile," 2008. National Adolescent Health Information Center, February 11, 2008, http://nahic.ucsf.edu/download/the-mental-health-of-adolescents-a-national-profile.

5. Centers for Disease Control and Prevention, "Youth Risk Behavior Surveillance System."

6. K. R. Puskar, L. Bernardo, M. Hatam, et al., "Self-Cutting Behaviors in Adolescents," *Journal of Emergency Nursing* 32, no. 5 (2006): 1–4.

7. Matt Walker, personal communication, March 16, 2012.

8. V. N. Salimpoor, M. Benovoy, K. Larcher, et al., "Anatomically Distinct Dopamine Release during Anticipation and Experience of Peak Emotion to Music," *Nature Neuroscience* 14 (2011): 257–62.

9. PHYSICAL WELLNESS

1. Dianne Neumark-Sztainer, *I'm, Like, SO Fat!: Helping Your Teen Make Healthy Choices about Eating and Exercise in a Weight-Obsessed World* (New York: Guilford, 2005).

2. Centers for Disease Control and Prevention, "Youth Risk Behavior Surveillance System: Selected 2011 National Health Risk Behaviors and Health Outcomes by Sex," 2011, www.cdc.gov/healthyyouth/yrbs/pdf/us_disparitysex_yrbs.pdf.

3. Ibid.

4. D. Neumark-Sztainer, M. E. Eisenberg, J. A. Fulkerson, et al., "Family Meals and Disordered Eating in Adolescents: Longitudinal Findings from Project EAT," *Archives of Pediatrics and Adolescent Medicine* 162, no. 1 (2008): 17–22.

5. Joel Fuhrman, phone interview on January 19, 2012.

6. Michael Holick, "Vitamin D Deficiency: Medical Progress," *New England Journal of Medicine* 357, no. 3 (2007): 266–281.

7. F. M. Gloth III, W. Alam, and B. Hollis, "Vitamin D vs Broad Spectrum Phototherapy in the Treatment of Seasonal Affective Disorder," *Journal of Nutrition, Health, and Aging* 3, no. 1 (1999): 5–7. Anna-Maija Tolppanen, Adrian Sayers, William D. Fraser, et al., "The Association of Serum 25-hydroxyvitamin D3 and D2 with Depressive Symptoms in Childhood—A Prospective Cohort Study," *Journal of Child Psychology and Psychiatry* 53, no. 1 (2012): 757–766.

8. Joel Fuhrman, *Eat to Live: The Amazing Nutrient-Rich Program for Fast and Sustained Weight Loss*. New York: Little, Brown, 2012.

9. Kathleen Zelman, "Clearing Up Confusion on Fats," United HealthCare, www.uhc.com/source4women/health_wellness_tools_resources/nutrition/confusion_on_fats.htm.

10. Jodi Greebel, phone interview, July 21, 2011.

11. C. A. Adebamowo, D. Spiegelman, C. S. Berkey, et al., "Milk Consumption and Acne in Adolescent Girls," *Dermatol Online Journal* 12 (2006): 1, http://dermatology.cdlib.org/124/original/acne/danby.html.

12. R. Smith, N. Mann, H. Makelainen, et al., "A Pilot Study to Determine the Short-Term Effects of a Low Glycemic Load Diet on Hormonal Markers of Acne: A Nonrandomized, Parallel, Controlled Feeding Trial," *Molecular Nutrition & Food Research* 52 (2008): 718–726.

13. R. Kaestner and X. Xu, "Effects of Title IX and Sports Participation on Girls' Physical Activity and Weight," *Advances in Health Economics and Health Services Research* 17 (2007): 79–111.

14. Luke M. Gessel, "Concussions among United States High School and Collegiate Athletes," *Journal of Athletic Training* 42, 4th ser. (2007): 495–503.

15. Michael Sokolove, "The Uneven Playing Field," *New York Times Magazine*, May 11, 2008, www.nytimes.com/2008/05/11/magazine/11Girls-t.html.

16. T. Covassin, R. J. Elbin, W. Harris, et al., "The Role of Age and Sex in Symptoms, Neurocognitive Performance, and Postural Stability in Athletes after Concussion," *American Journal of Sports Medicine* (2011): 1303–1312.

17. J. Gilchrist, B. R. Mandelbaum, H. Melancon, et al., "A Randomized Controlled Trial to Prevent Noncontact Anterior Cruciate Ligament Injury in Female Collegiate Soccer Players," *American Journal of Sports Medicine* 36, no. 8 (2008): 1476–1483.

18. Gretchen Reynolds, *The First 20 Minutes: Surprising Science Reveals How We Can Exercise Better, Train Smarter, Live Longer* (New York: Hudson Street Press, 2012), p. ix.

19. A. Woolery, H. Myers, B. Sternlieb, et al., "Yoga Intervention for Young Adults with

Elevated Symptoms of Depression," *Alternative Therapies in Health and Medicine* 10, no. 2 (2004): 60–63. M. Jaynbakht, R. Hejazi Kenari, M. Ghasemi, "Effects of Yoga on Depression and Anxiety of Women," *Complementary Therapies in Clinical Practice* 15, no. 2 (2009): 102–104.

10. SPIRITUAL WELLNESS

1. Alexandra Stoddard, *Things I Want My Daughters to Know* (New York: Willam Morrow, 2007), p. 102.

INDEX

|||||||||||||||||||||||||

Index

Index

Index

Index

Index

IIIIIIIIIIIIIIIIIIIIIIII

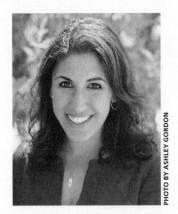

PHOTO BY ASHLEY GORDON

Ana Homayoun is the founder of Green Ivy Educational Consulting and the author of *That Crumpled Paper Was Due Last Week: Helping Disorganized and Distracted Boys Succeed in School and Life.* In addition to her individualized consulting services, Ana works internationally with students, parents, teachers, and school administrators on incorporating organization, time management, and personal purpose into the classroom and school culture. She is a frequent writer and speaker on adolescent and young adult issues, and consults with schools and organizations worldwide. A graduate of Duke University, she also holds a master's degree in counseling psychology and a Pupil Personnel Services credential. To learn more about Ana and her work, visit www.anahomayoun.com.